the

HERB

GARDENER'S

ESSENTIAL

GUIDE

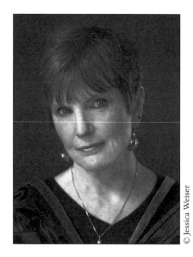

© Jessica Weiser

About the Author

Sandra Kynes is a yoga instructor, a Reiki practitioner, and a member of the Bards, Ovates and Druids. She likes developing creative ways to explore the world and integrating them with her spiritual path, which serves as the basis for her books. She has lived in New York City, Europe, England, and now coastal New England. She loves connecting with nature through gardening, hiking, and ocean kayaking. Visit her website at www.kynes.net.

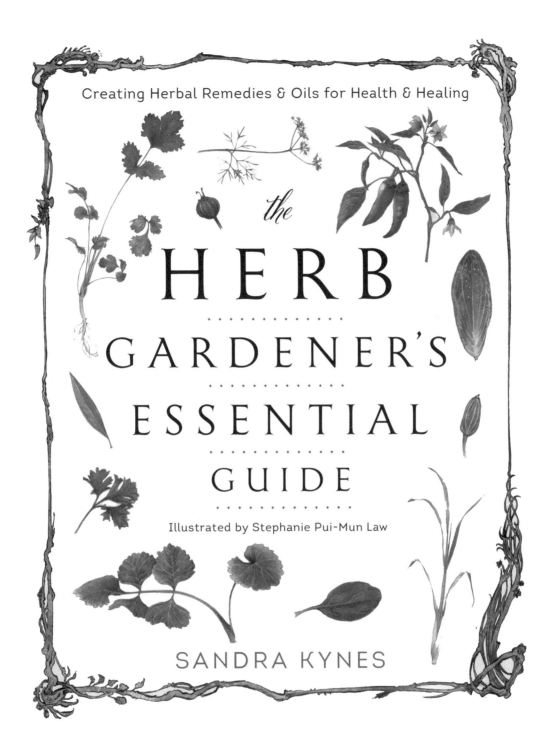

Creating Herbal Remedies & Oils for Health & Healing

the

HERB

· · · · · · · · · · ·

GARDENER'S

· · · · · · · · · · ·

ESSENTIAL

· · · · · · · · · · ·

GUIDE

· · · · · · · · · · ·

Illustrated by Stephanie Pui-Mun Law

SANDRA KYNES

Llewellyn Publications
Woodbury, Minnesota

First Edition
Second Printing, 2021

Book design and format: Donna Burch-Brown
Cover art: Stephanie Pui-Mun Law
Cover design: Kevin R. Brown
Editing: Stephanie Finne
Interior illustrations: Stephanie Pui-Mun Law and Llewellyn Art Department on pages 14, 15 and 38

Llewellyn Publishing is a registered trademark of Llewellyn Worldwide Ltd.

Library of Congress Cataloging-in-Publication Data
Kynes, Sandra, 1950–
  The herb gardener's essential guide : creating herbal remedies and oils for health & healing / by Sandra Kynes.
    pages cm
  Includes bibliographical references and index.
  ISBN 978-0-7387-4564-0
  1. Herbs—Therapeutic use. 2. Health. 3. Self-care, Health. I. Title.
  RM666.H33K96 2016
  615.3'21—dc23
                    2015015227

Llewellyn Publications
A Division of Llewellyn Worldwide Ltd.
2143 Wooddale Drive
Woodbury, MN 55125-2989
www.llewellyn.com

Printed in China

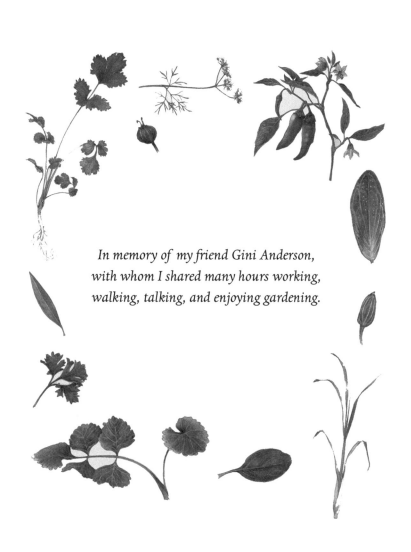

In memory of my friend Gini Anderson,
with whom I shared many hours working,
walking, talking, and enjoying gardening.

Acknowledgements

My thanks to Amy Glaser whose vision started this book,
Stephanie Pui-Mun Law for her beautiful artwork,
and Lynne Menturweck for her direction in pulling it all together;
Liz Parsons and Rosanne Graef for inviting me to join
our neighborhood apothecary garden project;
and my family Lyle Koehnlein and Jessica Weiser
who share a small oasis of a backyard garden with me.

Contents

INTRODUCTION

There is a special beauty to herbs. We may know many of them as unassuming garden plants, but their use is intertwined with human history. For thousands of years they have provided people with fragrance, taste, and healing. My interest in herbs has affected several aspects of my life—cooking, gardening, and the desire for natural healing—which has led to an interest in essential oils. Before going further, I must explain that I am not a trained herbalist nor am I certified through any program or school. I am like the many thousands throughout the ages who have gone before me to learn from others, observe, and study on my own. I grew up in a household where the first line of defense against illness or discomfort and the first aid rendered after injury came from the kitchen or my grandmother's garden. While commercial products eventually made their way into the medicine cabinet ("new" and "convenient" were the buzzwords of the early 1960s), my mother often drifted back to remedies she knew as a child. Because of that, I became familiar with them, too. However, while I consider herbs comforting, my preference for herbal remedies goes beyond childhood memories. Like many people today, I think nature offers a better way of dealing with common, basic health issues, and I prefer not to use medicines made from synthetic chemicals.

As I mentioned, I am not an expert. I work with herbs and essential oils for my own purposes and not to provide treatment to other people or sell products. While it may seem odd that I have written a book on herbs and essential oils, my purpose is to encourage others to explore the healthful bounty of the plant kingdom without feeling intimidated. After all, our ancestors were not "herbologists," they simply used the knowledge that was handed down through generations and did what they needed to do to relieve discomfort and stay healthy. That said, we must keep in mind that herbs are powerful and they must be used properly.

Like many books about herbs and healing remedies, details on how to grow and prepare them for use is also included here. However, I have veered onto my own path by integrating information on essential oils. After all, the history of essential oils is intertwined with that of herbal medicine. While essential oils require a great deal of plant material and few of us have the space to grow enough or the equipment to distill it, I have included them because they expand and enhance our herbal repertoire.

General Precautions

My purpose for writing this book is to encourage others to explore the health benefits of herbs without feeling intimidated, however, working with herbal remedies must be done with knowledge and common sense. Although herbs and essential oils are natural alternatives to synthetic, chemical-based remedies, they must be used with safety in mind. Herbs are powerful healers, but they can be harmful when not used properly.

If you have not used an herbal remedy before, start with a small amount to make sure you do not have an adverse reaction. If you have any sign of nausea, diarrhea, stomach upset, or headache discontinue use immediately. Herbal remedies are not recommended for internal use by children younger than two years old, and when given to an older child they should be diluted. Women who are pregnant or nursing must be sure to follow precautions carefully and are advised to consult their physician or specialist first. Anyone taking medications should also consult his or her doctor before using herbs, as they can interact with drugs.

In addition, it is important to work with your doctor when problems are prolonged or if they escalate. Luckily today more physicians are open to "alternative" treatments and working with their patients rather than dictating to them. While it may take time to find such a doctor, it is worth the effort.

How to Use This Book

Part 1 of this book provides details for creating and maintaining an apothecary garden as well as information for growing herbs in containers on a porch or a windowsill. If you have not gardened before, this part of the book will tell you how to plan your garden, the tools you'll need, how to get it started, and what you will need to be comfortable while working outside. In addition to general maintenance, you will learn what you need to do to tuck your plants in for the winter.

Part 2 provides instructions on how to harvest and preserve the parts of plants that you will need to create your own remedies. It is also a guide for making and using foundation mixtures such as infusions, decoctions, and tinctures. In addition, it provides details on how to make and use other forms of remedies, many of which are based on the foundation mixtures. You will also learn the basics about essential and carrier oils.

Part 3 of this book is an encyclopedic listing of twenty-eight herbs, which serves as a reference for their use as remedies. Each entry includes historical information about the plant, medicinal uses and recipes, along with precautions and contraindications. Information on using the essential oil is also included. For readers interested in gardening, there is a plant description with notes on growing it and harvesting its roots, stems, seeds, or flowers. Of course, each listing includes the plant's scientific name.

In conjunction with part 3, appendix A is a listing of ailments and conditions that provides a convenient cross-reference of remedies and herbs. Appendix B contains measurement equivalents to help you determine the easiest way to measure ingredients for your preparations.

Even if you have been gardening for years and/or making your own remedies, this book will serve as a handy reference for both herbs and essential oils to support your healing and good health.

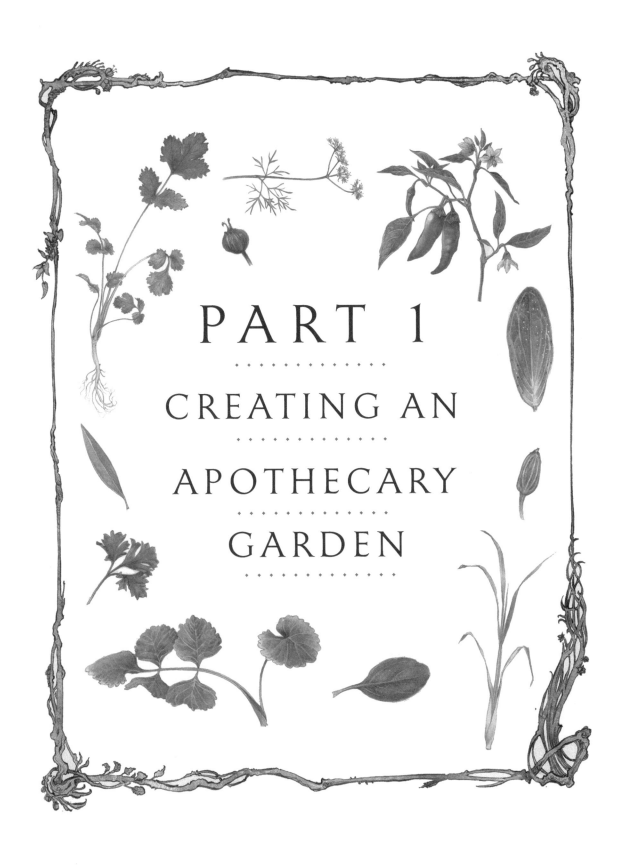

PART 1

· · · · · · ·

CREATING AN

· · · · · · · · ·

APOTHECARY

· · · · · · · · ·

GARDEN

· · · · · · · · ·

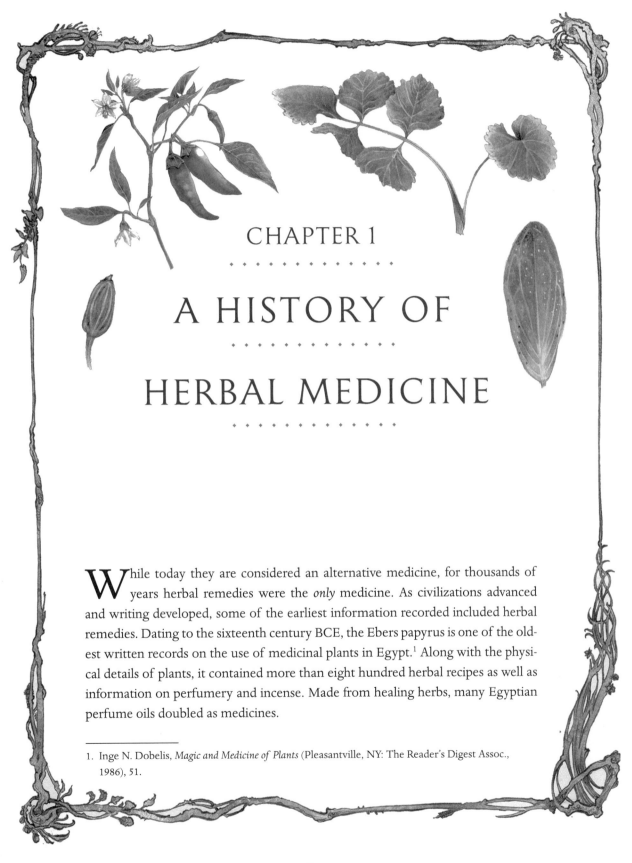

CHAPTER 1

· · · · · · · · · · · · · ·

A HISTORY OF

· · · · · · · · · · · · · ·

HERBAL MEDICINE

· · · · · · · · · · · · ·

While today they are considered an alternative medicine, for thousands of years herbal remedies were the *only* medicine. As civilizations advanced and writing developed, some of the earliest information recorded included herbal remedies. Dating to the sixteenth century BCE, the Ebers papyrus is one of the oldest written records on the use of medicinal plants in Egypt.[1] Along with the physical details of plants, it contained more than eight hundred herbal recipes as well as information on perfumery and incense. Made from healing herbs, many Egyptian perfume oils doubled as medicines.

---

1. Inge N. Dobelis, *Magic and Medicine of Plants* (Pleasantville, NY: The Reader's Digest Assoc., 1986), 51.

Some of the earliest writings from India contained information about herbs and spices. This evolved into Ayurvedic medicine, which is believed to be the oldest system of healing. Although the tenth-century Persian physician and philosopher Avicenna (980–1037) is often credited with discovering the distillation process, archaeological evidence suggests that distilling aromatic plants into oils was achieved in India around 3000 BCE.[2] Herbs are also integral to Traditional Chinese medicine, a system of healing that dates to approximately 200 BCE.

Known as *rhizotomoi*, "root gatherers," the herb merchants of ancient Greece kept records on the properties of herbs.[3] Greek physician Hippocrates (460–377 BCE), regarded as the "Father of Medicine," has been noted for his balanced, holistic approach, which included the use of herbal remedies. Several centuries later, Greek physician and botanist Pedanius Dioscorides (ca. 40–90 CE) compiled the first European manuscript on herbal remedies entitled *De Materia Medica*, "The Material of Medicine." As a prototype of the classical "herbal" on which our present-day books are patterned, it contained instructions for many types of preparations and served as a major reference book well into the seventeenth century.

Claudius Galenus better known as Galen (130–200 CE) was a prominent Roman physician whose writings included a range of herbal preparations. One of his elixirs, which became known as Venice Treacle, was popular into the eighteenth century.[4] Another influential writer was the Roman natural historian Pliny (23/24–79 CE). Eight of his thirty-seven books dealt with plant pharmacology and were a valuable resource for herbalists through the seventeenth century.

After the fall of the Roman Empire, Europe was plunged into the uncertainty of the Dark Ages. To escape the social upheaval, many physicians and other learned people relocated to Constantinople (now Istanbul, Turkey) and along with them went a storehouse of knowledge. However, even though European civilization floundered, the works of Hippocrates, Dioscorides, Pliny, and others were translated and widely distributed in the Middle East.

As life in Europe became more stable, scholars and medical knowledge filtered back and so too did the ancient texts of Greece, Rome, and Egypt. Tucked away in their monasteries, monks not only copied ancient books of remedies but also kept extensive herb gardens for culinary, healing, and religious purposes.

German abbess, writer, and mystic Hildegard of Bingen (1098–1179) was also a healer and an authority on herbs. She is the only medieval wisewoman whose work has survived. In contrast to the complicated formulas of others practicing medicine at that time, she relied on "simples," or preparations that used one herb rather than combinations of plants.

---

2. Julia Lawless, *The Illustrated Encyclopedia of Essential Oils: The Complete Guide to the Use of Oils in Aromatherapy and Herbalism* (London: Element Books, 1995), 18.

3. Barbara Griggs and Barbara Van der Zee, *Green Pharmacy: The History and Evolution of Western Herbal Medicine* (Rochester, VT: Healing Arts Press, 1997), 8.

4. Kate Kelly, *Early Civilizations: Prehistoric Times to 500 C.E.* (New York: Facts on File, 2009), 132.

The study that was taking place in monasteries sparked the creation of universities and medical schools. These schools played an important part in the development of the study of medicine. During this time, herbs were central to healing remedies. By the thirteenth century, the trade in herbs and spices expanded between the Middle East and Europe, and then to Asia and Africa. After Columbus's voyages, even more new medicinal plants arrived in Europe.

Despite this flood of plants and knowledge, many people did not have access to or could not afford doctor visits and remedies from exotic plants. Instead, they did what people had done for thousands of years and relied on local healers—the wisewomen who had special skills and knowledge.

A golden age of herbalism was sparked in the Elizabethan era by the use of the printing press. English physician and botanist John Gerard (1545–1612) was instrumental in introducing plants from the Americas to a wider audience in Europe. His work entitled *The Herball, or Generall Historie of Plantes* was published in 1597 and became a classic text. Physician and master herbalist Nicholas Culpeper (1616–1654) published his work entitled *The English Physitian* in 1653. This book has never gone out of print.

Even with the popular enthusiasm for herbals among lay people, change was in the air where the medical establishment was concerned. Seizing on the idea of Swiss physician Theophrastus von Hohenheim (1493–1541) that a little bit of something dangerous can be healing, conventional medicine separated paths with herbal-based remedies. Purging and bloodletting became popular treatments, as did the use of leeches. Anyone following folk traditions came to be regarded as amateurs, and herbal medicine was considered primitive and irrelevant. For a time, the use of herbs and oils was stifled by this schism, which was made worse by the waxing and waning hysteria over witchcraft. As a result, the village wisewomen suffered terribly.

Herbal remedies and perfumery eventually made a comeback as the world changed and attitudes shifted. Part of that shift was due to the Industrial Revolution, which sparked many new social developments. One was the creation of the suburbs. While suburban gardens were too small for the grand sprawling designs of the Renaissance, they were a good size for growing basic vegetables and herbs. Herbs and other plants found their way back into conventional medicine but mainly in research laboratories where the active components of plants were studied.

In the early twentieth century, the advancement of chemistry was not only overtaking the use of herbs and essential oils in medicines but in perfumes and cosmetics as well. French chemist René-Maurice Gattefossé (1881–1950) was responsible for resurrecting the use of essential oils during the 1920s. After burning his hand in his laboratory, he grabbed the nearest bottle of liquid, which turned out to be lavender oil. Intrigued by its rapid healing effect, he devoted the remainder of his career to studying essential oils. Although in the 1930s herbal remedies began to make a comeback in England, the 1940s ushered in an overwhelming amount of laboratory-produced medicine.

In Europe and the United States, the post-war shift toward the desire for things that were "new" (which equated to "better") regarded herbal remedies as outmoded. This was spurred on by a medical profession that considered the use of herbs as old-fashioned, superstitious belief. Once again, herbs were pushed out of medicine and this time from the garden, too. The new affluence and growth of the suburbs brought changes to how people used their outdoor space. Stretches of lawn became the norm with ornamental flower gardens for accent. Herbs were separated from decorative plants and relegated to their own little spot by the kitchen door, if they were grown at all.

The tide of public sentiment began to turn in the early 1960s with the thalidomide tragedy. Used to relieve morning sickness, the drug thalidomide caused a range of deformities in unborn babies. Faith in modern medicine was badly shaken and people's perceptions of drugs and health began to change.

Amidst the myriad of social changes during the 1960s, a back-to-the-land movement and the science of ecology emerged. With the growing awareness of how our health depends on the health of the planet, the genie was out of the bottle. Herbal medicine made a comeback and even the scientific community has begun to acknowledge its importance. Ironically, despite all the money spent on drug research and development, a substitute for digitalis (from the plant commonly known as foxglove, *Digitalis purpurea*) continues to elude production in the laboratory. In addition, scientists are wondering what undiscovered cures might come from unknown plants in places that have not been thoroughly explored, such as the Amazon River basin.

Although still considered "alternative" for the most part, the practice of Traditional Chinese and Ayurvedic medicines is increasing in Europe and the United States. In addition, growing herbs and using them medicinally is working its way into the mainstream as many of us take a more active role in our healing and well-being. As we do this, we come full circle to the wisewomen and men of the past who relished and relied on the herbal bounty of the earth.

Other Traditional Uses of Herbs

In addition to being an integral part of medicine and the culinary arts since ancient times, herbs have been important to a wider range of uses. While we have the convenience of ready-made products for everyday use, until the last century this was not the case and herbs were a major component of good housekeeping.

Used for laundering clothes and linens since Roman times, the name *lavender* comes from the Latin *lavare*, which means "to wash." The Old French word *lavanderie* means "laundry." [5] Along with lavender, other herbs such as rosemary, tansy, and woodruff were used in linen cupboards to keep away moths. Herbs were also used in the kitchen pantry to combat pests. Bay leaves placed in flour bins helped repel weevils, and tansy and rosemary rubbed on meat kept flies away. Sprigs of marjoram, mints, and pennyroyal were scattered on shelves to discourage ants.

Elsewhere in the house, herbs were used for cleaning and for odor and pest control. To avoid increasing dampness in a home during certain times of the year, fennel and mint were used to scrub

---

5. Ruth Binney, *The Gardener's Wise Words and Country Ways* (Newton Abbot, England: David and Charles, 2007), 126.

floors without water. Any bits of plant material left on the floor were simply swept up. Rosemary and lavender were also used for scrubbing floors in this manner. And for the furniture, lemon balm and marjoram were made into a polish. Herbs were also added to cushion and mattress stuffing for fragrance as well as to combat pests.

In Northern Europe and Britain from the Middle Ages to the late eighteenth century, strewing herbs was a vital part of good housekeeping. This practice of strewing plants on the floor helped to warm a house in the winter and cool it in the summer. It was common practice to spread rushes on earthen and stone floors with herbs such as savory and basil mixed in. Not only did this scent the air, the herbs acted as an antiseptic and aided in repelling fleas. Lavender and meadowsweet were used with reeds to overcome musty odors. Bunches of aromatic herbs were also hung about the house in the summer so the oxidizing essential oils could cool and refresh rooms. In the sixteenth century, violet, rosemary, and other distilled herbal waters were sprinkled on wooden floors to scent and cool rooms.

While the rich color purple used by royalty and high church officials was made from sea snails and prohibitively expensive, everyone else did not walk around in plain, drab clothes. A wide range of beautifully colored dyes were made from herbs. Yellows were created from chamomile, fennel, sage, St. John's wort, and yarrow; reds from dandelion, dock, and St. John's wort; blues from elder, indigo, and woad; greens from angelica, marjoram, and rosemary; and shades of gold from mullein and plantain.

In the past, herbs touched almost every aspect of everyday life. Now we are finding our way back to nature as many traditional herbal uses beyond healing remedies are being revived.

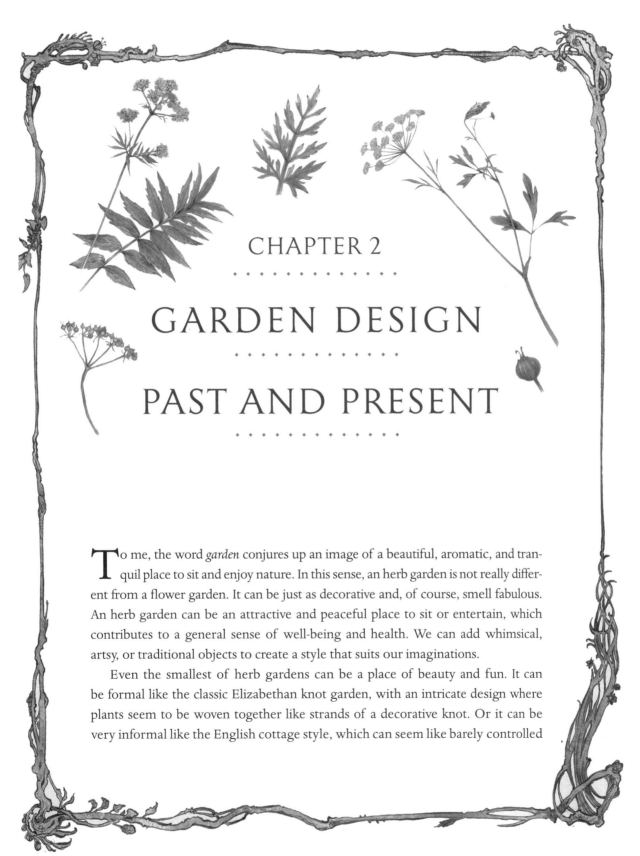

CHAPTER 2

GARDEN DESIGN

PAST AND PRESENT

To me, the word *garden* conjures up an image of a beautiful, aromatic, and tranquil place to sit and enjoy nature. In this sense, an herb garden is not really different from a flower garden. It can be just as decorative and, of course, smell fabulous. An herb garden can be an attractive and peaceful place to sit or entertain, which contributes to a general sense of well-being and health. We can add whimsical, artsy, or traditional objects to create a style that suits our imaginations.

Even the smallest of herb gardens can be a place of beauty and fun. It can be formal like the classic Elizabethan knot garden, with an intricate design where plants seem to be woven together like strands of a decorative knot. Or it can be very informal like the English cottage style, which can seem like barely controlled chaos. An herb garden can be modern, traditional, or themed just like a flower garden. It can also be a separate garden or an herb "room" (area) within a flower garden. In addition, herbs can be integrated into existing gardens of flowers, shrubs, or vegetables. In fact, herbs are very beneficial to other plants, which we will explore later, but first let's take a look at garden design.

The ancient Romans laid out their herb gardens in geometric patterns, making them practical and appealing. Medieval monastic gardens were rectangular with paths between rows of herbs and vegetables. Later, the artistic enthusiasm of the Renaissance extended to gardens. Geometric designs with squares and rectangles were worked into complex symmetrical patterns creating a living version of the Persian carpet. The Elizabethan era marked the dawn of extravagant pleasure gardens in royal courts as well as large estates. To disassociate their outdoor space from the cluttered appearance of cottager's gardens, the landed gentry kept their plants neatly trimmed and formal. This and the influence of popular Italian design resulted in the knot garden. While knot gardens are absolutely beautiful, they take more work to set up and the plants must be kept neatly clipped to maintain the appearance. That said, if it is the garden of your dreams, it is worth the effort.

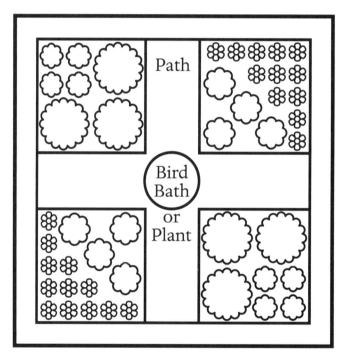

Figure 1.1. A formal look can be created by using geometric shapes with repeating form and color to unify the garden.

If a formal look appeals to you but you want a design that is less labor-intensive than a knot garden, the use of geometric patterns can help you achieve it. Geometric patterns can be created from a simple square-, rectangular-, or circular-shaped garden by putting paths between groups of plants. Paths can be created with gravel, stones, or bricks. Also, a traditional formal garden usually has something at the center to serve as a focal point. This can be a statue, gazing ball, potted plant, or anything that appeals to your sense of design. A birdbath works well, plus by inviting birds to your garden you are encouraging natural pest control.

A traditional informal design can be created by locating a garden along a wall or a fence with taller plants at the back and shorter ones in front. If you want to make an island and locate your garden in the middle of a lawn, arrange it with taller plants in the center and progressively shorter ones out to the edges. An island bed can be circular, oval, or kidney-shaped. It can also be a free-form garden with irregular, flowing borders. In addition, consider the shapes that can be created within the garden using plant colors and textures.

Layouts such as the ladder and cartwheel are popular designs for herb gardens. Bricks or small paving stones are often used to create the ladder rungs or wheel spokes. One type of herb is usually planted in each of the spaces.

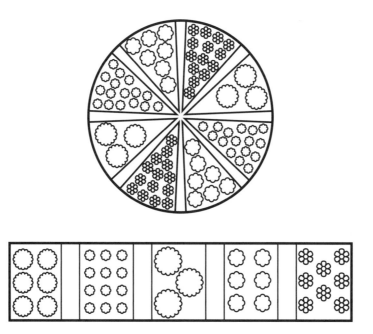

Figure 1.2. The wagon wheel and ladder design layouts are popular for herb gardens.

An important hallmark of good design for any type of garden is having the plants easy to reach. Not only does this make planting easier, but tasks such as weeding and harvesting can be done without trampling half the garden. If you don't want paths, a few flat stepping stones or bricks can be strategically placed to help you maneuver around the plants.

Another type of garden design is the raised bed, which has some advantages. In addition to being a solution for poor soil, it provides easy access to plants so you don't need to put in paths or do as much bending while working. It also provides good drainage. Raised beds allow you to accommodate the herbs you want to grow even if your soil is not what they require. Also, if you have more than one raised bed you can use different types of soil and group plants with similar requirements together. The gardening project at my neighborhood elementary school creatively uses raised beds by grouping them into geometric patterns.

The frames for raised beds can be built with wood, bricks, or stones. If you make your own with wood, purchase the type that is untreated so chemicals won't leach into the soil. Ready-made frames are also available. Once the frames are up it is easy to get started: pour in bagged soil, work in some compost, and you are ready to plant. My son and I used a raised bed to solve a landscape problem with our backyard. The property behind ours is a few feet higher and our yard sloped directly toward the house. To ease the slope, we installed a raised bed along the back fence by stacking long, heavy timbers to create a terrace. To keep the timbers aligned, my son connected them with long, thick screws. This terrace measures about two feet from front to back and creates a perfect border garden because it is easy to work in.

Don't be shy about integrating herbs into your current landscaping. Bushy lavender plants can set off a path or highlight a decorative fence, and Roman chamomile can be used for ground cover in partially shaded areas. Also, herbs such as lemon balm and chervil can thrive in moderately moist areas where other plants may not fare as well.

Amongst the stones or bricks of paths and patios, low-growing herbs can enhance the stonework and help keep weeds at bay. A patio is a particularly good place for herbs because it is usually situated in a sunny location. Aromatic herbs will warm with the stonework and scent the air, creating a pleasant outdoor space. Creeping thyme and Roman chamomile work well for this.

As previously mentioned, herbs can be integrated into an established garden of vegetables, shrubs, and flowers. They can enhance the colors and scent of a garden, too. Also, many herbs are helpful in the vegetable garden as companion plants that attract beneficial insects and deter the bad ones.

Location, Location, Location

Now that you may have some creative ideas for your herb garden, it's time to start the practical planning. If you are starting a garden from scratch, the first step is to figure out the best location for it. Go outside several times on the same day and take a look at your property. Note where is it sunny or shady. From memory, or over the course of several months, note from which direction your property gets the most wind and where frost or snow lingers. In addition, take note of areas where water may puddle. Also find out where water lines, electrical cables, septic tanks, or underground oil tanks may be buried. It's not that you will be digging really deep, but keep in mind that when these services need repair or replacement, your garden will become a casualty. If possible, consider positioning the garden where you can see it from a window to extend your enjoyment of it.

Even if you are adding herbs to an existing garden, you will want to do some assessment. Check if the plants you already have could benefit from the herbs you are interested in growing and group them accordingly. And remember the importance of having planting areas that are easy to get at and work in. While the stars don't always perfectly align to give us the best of everything, with some planning and ingenuity we can create a garden that suits our tastes and accommodates the plants' requirements.

Why Scientific Names Are Important

While the common names for plants are easy to remember, they are a source of confusion because one plant may be known by a number of names. For example, the flower widely known as bleeding heart (*Lamprocapnos spectabilis* syn. *Dicentra spectabilis*) is also known as Dutchman's trousers, lady in a bath, and lyre flower. And the blue flag (*Iris versicolor*) is also known as the northern blue flag, flag lily, and water lily. For this reason, it is important to know the scientific (genus and species) names when purchasing seeds, herbs, and essential oils. This way, you will be sure of getting the right ones.

Genus and species are part of a complex naming structure initiated by Swedish naturalist Carl Linnaeus (1707–1778). His work became the foundation for the International Code of Botanical Nomenclature. Over time, as new knowledge about plants emerged, their names were changed to reflect the new data. This is one reason why we find synonyms in botanical names. Antiquated names are kept to aid in identification, as in the example of the bleeding heart above. Another reason is scientific disagreement.

Most names are in Latin because during Linnaeus's time Latin was a common language that people engaged in scientific research could share. The first of the two words in the scientific name is the genus, which is a proper noun and always capitalized. A plant's species name is an adjective that usually provides a little description about the plant. The genus for yarrow is *Achillea* in honor of the Greek hero Achilles, and the species that is included in this book is *millefolium*. The word *millefolium* indicates a leaf of many parts (*mille* meaning "thousands" and *folium* meaning "foliage"). Occasionally you may see a third word in a name preceded with "var." indicating that it is a variety of that species. For example, the naturally occurring white-flowered rosemary has the scientific name of *Rosmarinus officinalis* var. *albiflorus*. Sometimes a variety is referred to as a subspecies, however, this term is often regarded as a gray area.

A third word may also indicate a cultivar, or more appropriately, a cultivated variety. This type of plant was created in the garden and not found naturally in the wild. The cultivar name is written in single quotes. For example, *Mentha spicata* 'Kentucky Colonel' is a cultivated variety of spearmint. The more modern cultivar names are written in English instead of Latin. You may also see an "x" in a name and this indicates that the plant is a hybrid. *Mentha x piperita*, peppermint, is a naturally occurring hybrid between spearmint, *Mentha spicata*, and water mint, *Mentha aquatica*.

Following the two- or three-word name you may also see a letter or sometimes a name, which identifies the individual who named the plant. For example, an "L." following a plant name means that it was bestowed by Linnaeus himself.

While it is not necessary to memorize the scientific names of the herbs with which you want to work, it is a good idea to jot them down to take with you when you go shopping for plants or essential oils. This way you can be sure to get the correct ones.

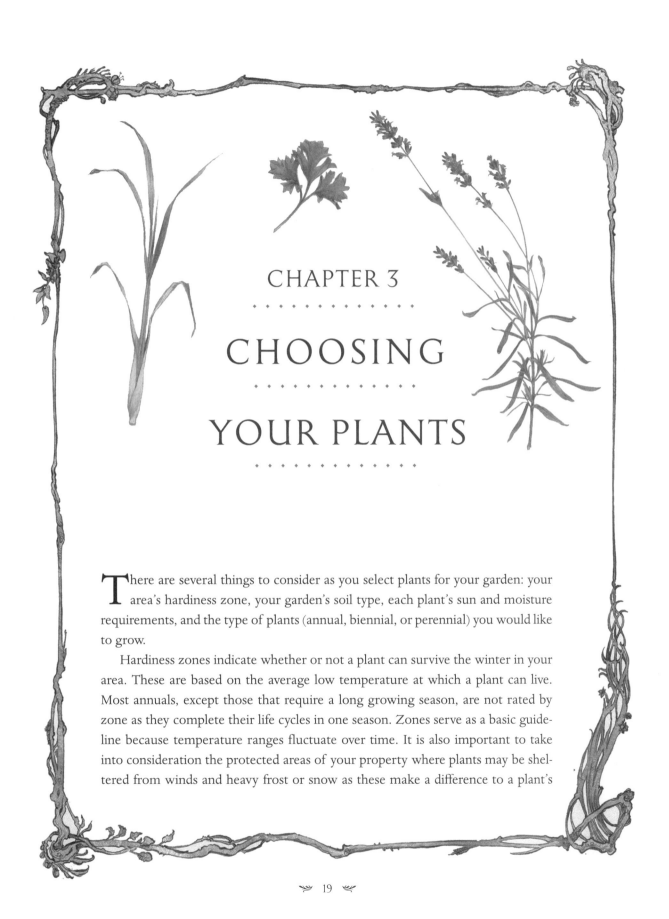

CHAPTER 3

· · · · · · · · ·

CHOOSING

· · · · · · · · ·

YOUR PLANTS

· · · · · · · · ·

There are several things to consider as you select plants for your garden: your area's hardiness zone, your garden's soil type, each plant's sun and moisture requirements, and the type of plants (annual, biennial, or perennial) you would like to grow.

Hardiness zones indicate whether or not a plant can survive the winter in your area. These are based on the average low temperature at which a plant can live. Most annuals, except those that require a long growing season, are not rated by zone as they complete their life cycles in one season. Zones serve as a basic guideline because temperature ranges fluctuate over time. It is also important to take into consideration the protected areas of your property where plants may be sheltered from winds and heavy frost or snow as these make a difference to a plant's survivability. Refer to the map in Figure 1.3 to help you determine which plants may work best in your area. More detailed and regional maps from the United States Department of Agriculture (USDA) can be found online.[6]

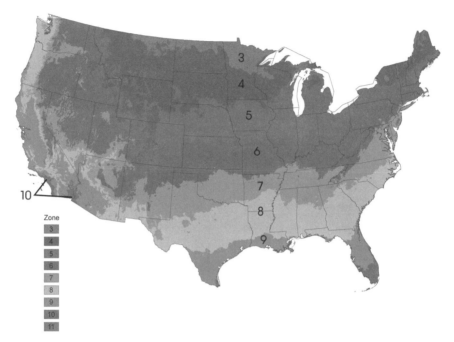

Figure 1.3. This is one of many plant hardiness zone maps provided by the US Department of Agriculture.

I live in zone 5 of northern New England, so a plant that is hardy to zone 8, the southern states, is not going to survive in my backyard. However, a plant designated as zone 6 may grow in my garden if it is in a sheltered location. Sometimes it is worth experimenting. A technique to try for plants of a warmer zone than where you live is called "over-wintering," which is easier to do with plants that are kept in containers. It simply requires that the plant be moved to a warmer, usually indoor, location during the winter. One that I want to try is rosemary. This shrubby evergreen is hardy to zone 7 and obviously will not survive outdoors in a Maine winter. However, with the right conditions indoors, it might do well.

Soil type is the next factor to consider when choosing plants. There are many ways that soil is described, such as light or heavy, but these terms are not all that helpful. Also, while some sources may list up to ten, there are really just four basic types of soil: sandy, silt, clay, and loam. An easy way to figure out what you have is to fill a jar with soil from your garden. Put the lid on tight, shake

6. Visit http://plalnthardiness.ars.usda.gov for more USDA maps.

it vigorously, and then let it sit for a day or two. The soil will settle into distinct layers. With larger particles, sand will settle to the bottom, clay will go to the top, and silt will be in-between. Their percentages will indicate the type of soil you have. If there is a fairly even amount of all three, your soil is called loam.

While a loam soil is considered the best for general gardening, the other types can be adjusted with compost (see chapter 7). When plant guidelines call for rich soil, it is referring to a loamy soil that has been well composted or fertilized. If you want to grow plants that require sandy soil but your garden is mostly clay, do not add only sand as you will end up with a sort of concrete. Use compost and a little sand to condition a clay soil. Soil type can also be dealt with by using raised beds, containers, or a combination of these.

Along with soil type, moisture content is something to keep in mind when planning which plants to group. An herb that needs dry conditions should not be planted with ones requiring higher moisture. Also, keep in mind that the term "moist soil" does not mean that it should be soggy or waterlogged.

Soil Type and Moisture Content	
Basic Soil Types	
Sandy	Largest particles, dry and gritty to the touch, does not hold water
Silt	Medium-size particles, smooth to the touch, slick when wet
Clay	Smallest particles, smooth to the touch when dry, sticky when wet
Loam	A mix of sand, silt, and clay
Soil Moisture Content	
Dry	Limited watering, soil dry to the touch even below the surface
Moderately dry	Top of soil is dry to the touch but may be slightly damp underneath
Moderately moist	Top of soil may be slightly dry to the touch but remains a little damp underneath
Moist	Needs frequent watering, soil remains moist to the touch, should never dry out, should not become a puddle or waterlogged

Sun requirements are, of course, an important consideration, too. Here again, the requirement categories are basic guidelines. I have found that some plants noted to require full sun actually do well in the parts of my garden that do not get a full six hours of direct sunlight. However, these areas are sheltered by a fence and I think the warmth that is maintained in these locations provides a good balance. Experimentation is the best way to determine what will work best for your garden.

Sun Requirements Decoded	
Full sun	At least 6 hours of direct sun
Partial sun	Between 4 to 6 hours of sun
Partial shade	Between 2 to 4 hours of sun. While plants in this category need sun, they also need relief from it.
Shade	Less than 2 hours of direct sun
Dappled or filtered sun	A mix of sun and shade

Don't let all this information overwhelm you. Knowing the conditions in your garden allows you to choose the most appropriate plants. Refer to the Plants at a Glance table for an overview of the general requirements for the herbs listed in part 3 of this book. While we want to provide the best conditions for our plants, one of the good things about herbs is that they are generally hardy and can do well even if everything is not perfect.

Another point to consider is the types of plants you want to grow. Like flowers, herbs fall into the categories of annuals, biennials, and perennials. As its name implies, an annual completes its life cycle in one year. It flowers, sets seed, and dies in a single season. Biennials take two seasons. These usually only bloom and set seed in their second season. Perennials live from year to year. While the top portion usually dies back in the autumn, the roots remain alive but dormant through winter. In the spring, perennials come up again.

Annuals take a little more work, as they need to be replaced each year. Some will reseed themselves, but not all. One thing I enjoy about annuals is the change-up they give to my garden each season. They can be grouped differently and planted in different spots. In addition, even though biennials have longer lifetimes, they can be changed out every couple of years for different effects.

You should also consider the remedies you want to make when choosing plants. For example, if you and your family are prone to catching colds and the flu or suffer from digestive issues, you may want to consider a garden that will be most useful for these particular needs. Appendix A will be helpful for this as it contains a listing of ailments and conditions and the herbs used to treat them.

Plants at a Glance							
Herb	*Type*	*Zone*	*Light*	*Soil*	*Moisture*	*Height*	*Spacing*
Angelica	Biennial	4	Partial shade	Loam	Moderately moist	5–8'	3'
Anise	Annual	Any	Full sun	Sandy loam	Dry	24"	12–18"
Basil	Annual	Any	Full sun	Loam	Moist	1–2'	12–18"

Plants at a Glance (cont.)							
Herb	*Type*	*Zone*	*Light*	*Soil*	*Moisture*	*Height*	*Spacing*
Bay	Perennial	8	Full sun to partial shade	Sandy loam	Moderately dry	2–50'	Depends on pruning
Borage	Annual	Any	Full sun	Sandy or chalky loam	Moist	1–3'	24"
Caraway	Biennial	3	Full sun	Sandy loam	Slightly dry	18–24"	6–8"
Cayenne	Annual	7	Full sun	Any	Moist	24–36"	24"
German chamomile	Annual	Any	Full sun to partial shade	Sandy	Moderately dry	30"	6–8"
Roman chamomile	Perennial	5	Partial shade	Loam	Moderately moist	8–9"	18"
Clary	Biennial	4	Full sun	Slightly sandy loam	Moderately moist	2–3'	9–12"
Coriander/ cilantro	Annual	Any	Full sun to partial shade	Any	Dry	18–14"	8–10"
Dill	Annual	Any	Full sun	Loam	Average moisture	3'	10–12"
Fennel	Perennial	4	Full sun	Sandy or loam	Moderately dry	4–5'	12"
Garlic	Perennial	4	Full sun	Loam	Moderately moist	1–2'	6"
Hyssop	Perennial	4	Full sun to partial shade	Sandy or loam	Moderately dry	2'	12"
Lavender	Perennial	5	Full sun to partial shade	Slightly sandy loam	Dry	2–3'	12–24"
Lemon balm	Perennial	4	Full sun to partial shade	Loam or sandy loam	Moderately moist	1–3'	12–24"
Lemongrass	Perennial	9	Full sun	Sandy loam	Moist	3–5'	2–4"
Marjoram	Perennial	9	Full sun	Sandy	Moderately dry	12"	6–8"

Plants at a Glance (cont.)							
Herb	*Type*	*Zone*	*Light*	*Soil*	*Moisture*	*Height*	*Spacing*
Parsley	Biennial	5	Full sun to partial shade	Loam	Moist	12"	8–10"
Peppermint	Perennial	5	Full sun to partial shade	Loam or slight clay	Moist	12–36"	12–24"
Rosemary	Perennial	8	Full sun	Sandy	Dry	3–6'	24–36"
Sage	Perennial	4	Full sun to partial shade	Sandy loam	Moderately moist	1–3'	24"
St. John's wort	Perennial	3	Full sun to partial shade	Slightly sandy loam	Moderately dry	2–3'	16–18"
Spearmint	Perennial	4	Partial shade	Loam	Moist	12–18"	12–24"
Thyme	Perennial	5	Full sun to partial shade	Sandy loam	Moderately dry	6–12"	10–12"
Valerian	Perennial	4	Partial shade to full sun	Loam	Moist	3–5'	36"
Yarrow	Perennial	2	Full sun to partial shade	Any	Moist	1–3'	18"

Depending on the herb and the part or parts of it that you want to use to make remedies, you may need more than one plant. This is because most leaves are better when they are harvested before a plant flowers. For example, if you want to use the leaves, seeds, and roots of angelica you will need separate plants. On the plant from which you take leaves, cut the flower heads off so they do not bloom and go to seed. This way, you can continue harvesting leaves that will be full of flavor and medicinal potency. The plants that you let flower are the ones from which you would harvest seeds and roots. Sow a few of the seeds in the autumn to propagate more plants. Angelica is a biennial that is good at reseeding itself. I started out with two small plants and now have an angelica patch in a corner of my garden.

Plan for Aggressive Plants

Peppermint and spearmint have robust root systems that can be invasive and take over your garden. The easiest way to deal with them is to grow them in containers. Another way to keep them in check is to sink barriers about twelve inches deep into the soil around them. Stones, bricks, or other garden edging material can be used for the barriers. Large clay flowerpots or clay chimney flues also work well. In addition, the roots of marjoram can become aggressive if the plant is not divided every couple of years.

Given a chance, dill, lemon balm, St. John's wort, and valerian will also try to take over the garden, but not because of rambunctious root systems. You can almost guarantee that any seeds they drop will sprout, producing many plants. This can be avoided by removing the flowers before they have a chance to go to seed. You will find more information about growing herbs in containers in chapter 9.

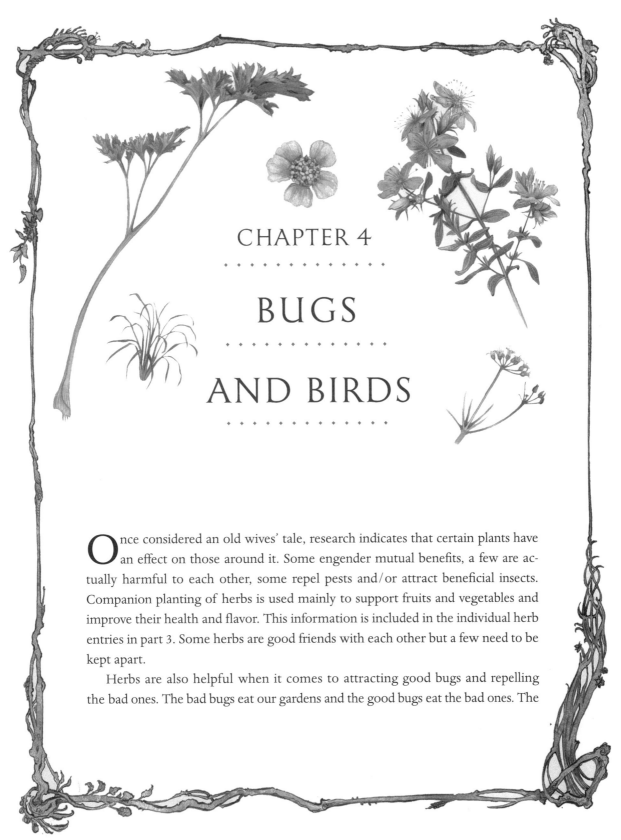

CHAPTER 4

· · · · · · · · · · · · · · ·

BUGS

· · · · · · · · · · · · · · ·

AND BIRDS

· · · · · · · · · · · · · · ·

Once considered an old wives' tale, research indicates that certain plants have an effect on those around it. Some engender mutual benefits, a few are actually harmful to each other, some repel pests and/or attract beneficial insects. Companion planting of herbs is used mainly to support fruits and vegetables and improve their health and flavor. This information is included in the individual herb entries in part 3. Some herbs are good friends with each other but a few need to be kept apart.

Herbs are also helpful when it comes to attracting good bugs and repelling the bad ones. The bad bugs eat our gardens and the good bugs eat the bad ones. The

Companion Planting and Bugs table provides information on how the herbs included in this book affect other plants. The table also includes details on some of the insects the herbs in this book attract or repel. The Good Bugs table provides details on the good bugs.

Bugs: Friend or Foe

An age-old method for thwarting the bad bugs is straightforward and simple: plant a variety of herbs. It doesn't have to be a wide variety of different plants, just avoid having a lot of one type of herb so pests won't be attracted by a large target.

It also helps to grow annuals in a different spot each year and transplant perennials every four to six years. Since pests usually need more than one season to establish themselves, changing the plants around disrupts them. In addition to weeding and keeping the garden cleaned up, composting to keep the soil healthy encourages beneficial organisms, which will help keep the bad ones in check.

Companion Planting and Bugs			
Herb	*Good For*	*Bad For*	*Bugs*
Anise	Coriander/cilantro; cabbage	Carrots	Repels cabbage loopers, imported cabbage moths
Basil	Peppers, tomatoes		Repels asparagus beetles, fleas, flies, mosquitoes
Bay			Repels weevils
Borage	Beans, cucumbers, strawberries, tomatoes		Attracts bees; repels tomato hornworms
Caraway	Peas		
Cayenne	Cucumbers, eggplants, tomatoes		Repels moths, weevils
Chamomile, German	Most herbs, especially basil, dill, peppermint; cabbage, cucumbers, onions		Attracts predatory wasps, hoverflies; repels fleas
Chamomile, Roman	Most herbs, especially basil, dill, peppermint		Attracts predatory wasps, hoverflies; repels fleas
Clary			Attracts bees
Coriander/ Cilantro	Anise, caraway; spinach	Fennel	Attracts bees; repels aphids, beetles, spider mites
Dill	Cabbage, corn, cucumbers, lettuce, onions	Fennel; carrots, tomatoes	Attracts bees; repels cabbage loopers, cabbage moths, tomato hornworms

Herb	Good For	Bad For	Bugs
\multicolumn{4}{c}{Companion Planting and Bugs (cont.)}
Fennel		Most especially caraway and dill; bush beans, kohlrabi, tomatoes	Attracts ladybugs; repels aphids, slugs, snails
Garlic	Cabbage, celery, cucumbers, eggplants, fruit trees, lettuce, peas, roses, tomatoes		Attracts butterflies; repels ants, aphids, Japanese beetles, slugs, snails
Hyssop	Cabbage, grapes		Attracts bees, butterflies; repels beetles, cabbage loopers, imported cabbage moths, fleas
Lavender	Yarrow; daylilies, dianthus, coreopsis, yucca		Attracts bees, butterflies
Lemon Balm	Pumpkins, squash		Attracts bees; repels squash bugs
Lemongrass	Lavender, mints, sage		Repels ants, flies, mosquitoes
Marjoram	Asparagus, beets, corn, cucumbers, lettuce, onions, peas, potatoes, squash, tomatoes, zucchini		Repels ants
Parsley	Most vegetables		
Peppermint	Cayenne, chamomile; cabbage, tomatoes	Parsley	Attracts hoverflies, predatory wasps; repels ants, aphids, bees, flea beetles, white cabbage moths
Rosemary	Sage; beans, cabbage		Attracts bees; repels bean beetles, cabbage flies, slugs, snails
Sage	Marjoram, rosemary; beans, cabbage, carrots, strawberries, tomatoes	Onions	Attracts bees, butterflies; repels cabbage loopers, carrot rust flies, imported cabbage moths
Spearmint	Cabbage, tomatoes	Parsley	Attracts hoverflies, predatory wasps; repels ants, aphids, flea beetles, white cabbage moths

Companion Planting and Bugs (cont.)			
Herb	*Good For*	*Bad For*	*Bugs*
Thyme	Eggplants, potatoes, tomatoes		Attracts bees; repels cabbage worms, whiteflies
Valerian	Most vegetables		Attracts bees, butterflies
Yarrow	Most aromatic herbs		Attracts ladybugs, hoverflies, and predatory wasps

The Good Bugs	
Bugs	*Benefits*
Bumblebees and honeybees	The best pollinators
Butterflies	Aid in pollination
Damselflies	Destroy aphids and a range of other bad bugs
Dragonflies	Destroy flies and mosquitoes
Ground beetles	Destroy cutworms, gypsy moth larvae, and root maggots
Hoverflies	Destroy aphids
Lacewings	Destroy aphids and other bad bugs
Ladybugs	Destroy aphids, mealy bugs, and mites
Praying mantis	Destroy a wide range of bad bugs
Spiders	Destroy a range of bad bugs
Wasps	Small parasitic wasps destroy aphids and caterpillars; the larger predatory wasps destroy caterpillars, and grubs; wasps are also good pollinators

Birds: The Gardener's Allies

Attracting birds to our backyards provides natural pest control for our gardens. While we might think of putting out a bird feeder only in the winter, birds can use help all year round because of diminishing habitats. The food in the feeder will attract birds but most of them eat a combination of insects, berries, and seeds, so after dining on what you provide they usually stick around to see what else they may find. Year-round residents that stake out your yard as a good food source will also attract migrating birds.

Feeding in the spring is especially important for the birds returning to your area until they reestablish the lay of the land for multiple feeding sites. While summer offers abundant natural sources for food, extra help filling the mouths of hatchlings is a big attraction for busy parent birds. In the autumn, migrating birds need to get ready for their long journeys, and of course, winter is most important when natural sources really dwindle.

In addition to food, providing water for birds is another good way to attract them to your yard. A birdbath can also function as a decorative feature and a focal point for your garden. Instead of a birdbath, use a large flowerpot saucer on the ground or on an up-ended flowerpot in the garden. If your porch is your garden, place a saucer amongst the containers. Feeders and birdbaths should be located near vegetation, which provides birds a safe place to wait their turn at the feeder or to take cover from a predator. Also, it is important to keep feeders and baths clean to avoid diseases.

Another attraction is to simply leave an area of your yard as natural as possible. This can be just some leaf litter under a shrub, which will encourage birds to forage for insects. A bare patch of loose soil will also appeal to birds for taking dust baths. In addition to keeping insects in check, some birds, such as finches and sparrows, are helpful for weed control because they have a fondness for many types of weed seeds.

The availability of nesting sites also lures birds. Trees and shrubs offer natural places but we can foster their interest by providing nest boxes or birdhouses. Ideally, these should be at least five feet above the ground, out of direct sunlight, and sheltered from heavy rain. Locating these near trees or shrubs is helpful. An exception is a martin house, which should be pole mounted about fourteen feet above the ground and at least fifteen feet away from structures. Martins like to be able to circle their colonies. There are two excellent websites for more information about attracting birds to your backyard: the Cornell Lab of Ornithology at www.allaboutbirds.org and the Audubon Society at www.audubon.org. In addition, consider putting up a bat box to provide a nearby roost. Bats are excellent helpers for insect control.

Inviting birds to your backyard will not completely rid your garden of insects but they will help maintain a healthy, balanced environment free of pesticides. Of course, there are other benefits beyond gardening. Bird watching is a relaxing pastime and a good stress-buster. It is also a fun, educational experience to share with children.

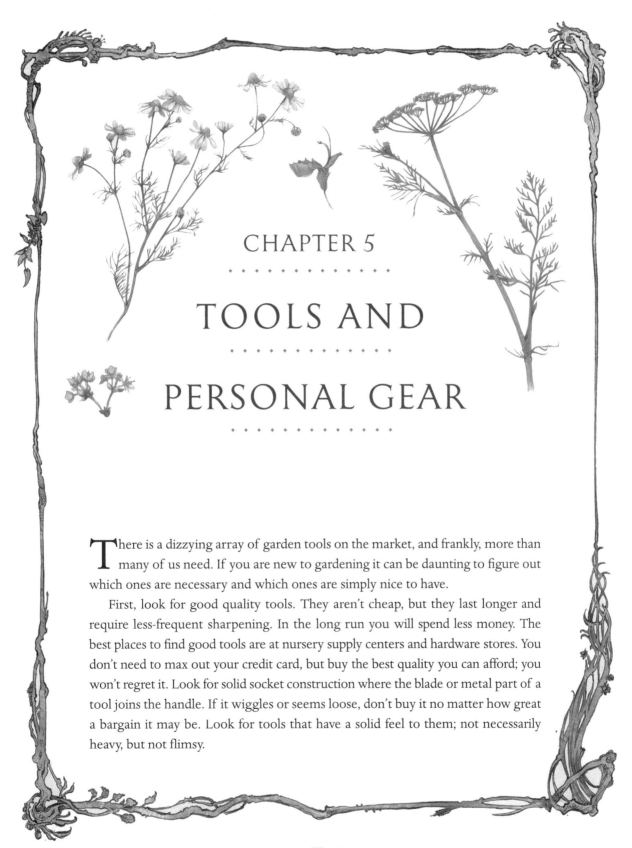

CHAPTER 5

· · · · · · · · · · ·

TOOLS AND

· · · · · · · · · · ·

PERSONAL GEAR

· · · · · · · · · · ·

There is a dizzying array of garden tools on the market, and frankly, more than many of us need. If you are new to gardening it can be daunting to figure out which ones are necessary and which ones are simply nice to have.

First, look for good quality tools. They aren't cheap, but they last longer and require less-frequent sharpening. In the long run you will spend less money. The best places to find good tools are at nursery supply centers and hardware stores. You don't need to max out your credit card, but buy the best quality you can afford; you won't regret it. Look for solid socket construction where the blade or metal part of a tool joins the handle. If it wiggles or seems loose, don't buy it no matter how great a bargain it may be. Look for tools that have a solid feel to them; not necessarily heavy, but not flimsy.

Take your time when you go to buy tools. Pick up different ones to see how they feel in your hand. Experiment with the motions that you will use in the garden. A tool that feels too big or heavy will be less effective if it causes your hand or arm to tire quickly. Don't be embarrassed or feel silly for doing this in the store, if anything it will make you look like an expert even if these are your first gardening tools. The following tools and equipment will help you handle all the basic tasks and more.

Shovel: The most useful type of shovel is a combination of shovel and spade. The garden spade is designed for digging into and loosening soil. It has a narrow, flat blade that is usually rectangular in shape with a rolled top edge. A shovel is wider, slightly concave, and designed for moving loose material around. The bottom edge of the blade is rounded to a center point. A combination shovel does both jobs. The blade of the combination shovel is wider than a spade and just concave enough for picking up material. The bottom edge is like a shovel and rounded to a center point. Like a spade, the top of the blade is rolled so you can comfortably place your foot on it and use your weight when necessary for digging. These shovels are available with either a short or a long handle to accommodate people of different heights. Use one with a handle length that will allow you to work without straining your back.

Level-head rake: This type of rake has short metal tines for dealing with material heavier than leaves. The tines are spaced wider apart than a leaf rake. The level-head rake is great for leveling soil, working with mulch, and post-season clean up.

Trowel: This hand tool is indispensable. It looks like a little shovel and is used for digging small holes and breaking up the soil. Like the shovel, there are many types of trowels. The most versatile have a pointed, slightly concave blade. Quality is especially important because the shovel blades of cheap trowels are easily bent. In addition, some trowels have a measurement scale on the blade, which is handy for getting the right depth when planting seeds and bulbs. The trowel is my most-used tool.

Hand rake: Also called a hand cultivator, this tool looks like a claw. It usually has three widely-spaced, curved tines and a short handle. It is good for weeding and keeping the soil loose around the base of plants.

Spading fork: Also called a garden fork, it has four long, strong tines that end in sharp points. It is used for digging and loosening soil, and it is especially useful when dividing the roots of plants for propagation. The spading fork differs from a pitchfork in that its tines are thicker, stronger, and spaced closer together.

Pruning clippers: These are also called pruning shears, hand pruners, and secateurs. They are best described as a type of scissors. Hand pruners have a short, curved blade that is good for cutting stems and branches. While this tool may get a lot more use at harvest time, it is handy for general maintenance throughout the season. There are pruners designed for lefties, too.

Grass shears: These are handy to keep the grass edging neat if your garden borders a lawn because you don't want to get too close to your herbs with a lawn mower. There are two types of shears: vertical and horizontal, which describes the direction the blades open. Some have a swivel mechanism that allows them to open either way. I find the horizontal easier to use.

Knives, scissors, and a teaspoon: A paring knife or a pair of scissors is handy for opening bags and seed packets. A sturdy old butter knife from the kitchen works well to dig holes when planting seeds and sometimes for weeding. Also raid the kitchen for an old teaspoon, which is helpful when handling seedlings.

Baskets or buckets: It is helpful to have three of these in your gear. Use one to hold your small tools so they are easier to move around the garden as you work. Use another to hold pulled weeds. The third may not be needed until the growing season is well under way, but it's good to have it handy for flowers or leaves that may be ready for harvesting during the summer.

Watering can: Whether or not you have a garden hose, this is better for watering seedlings and small, delicate plants when they are first put in the garden. The type of spout nozzle called a "rose" has a wide, flat cover with holes that separate the stream of water and helps to moisten plants more evenly. Using a watering can instead of a hose also makes it easier to take care of plants with slightly different moisture requirements because you can selectively water them.

When you are using tools in the garden, be mindful of where you set them down. A rake left on the ground with the tines pointing up becomes a serious hazard should someone step on it. Unfortunately, I speak from experience, having stepped on a rake that I left on the ground. When you are finished working for the day, brush away any soil on the tools and wipe them off with a rag or a paper towel. Taking care of your tools will help them last longer. Store them in a convenient place and keep sharp ones out of the reach of small children.

Personal Gear: Be Prepared, Be Comfortable

When gardening, it is important to be comfortable and protected. Because getting dirty and sweaty is part of the process, it's a good idea to wear old clothes and shoes. If you are clearing an area for your garden, you may want to wear long pants and sleeves for protection. Also, choose clothing that allows you to move freely. Old sneakers or hiking boots are comfortable choices for foot gear. Remember, you are working with tools and need to protect your feet. When first starting your garden, boots are better as you will be using your feet on a shovel to dig and a boot makes it easier than a sneaker. If your backyard has uneven terrain, as mine does, sturdy footwear can help prevent falls or twisted ankles. Flip-flops are fine when weeding and doing light tasks, but they are not a good choice when digging and raking.

Garden gloves are essential. They save a lot of wear and tear on the hands, especially fingernails and fingertips. Gloves help avoid blisters and protect you from poison ivy, thorns, startled spiders that may bite, or other creepy-crawlies that may not like your presence. Get a pair that fit comfortably and do not feel clumsy. If you need to work in wet soil, a pair of rubber kitchen gloves works nicely.

There are a few other things that will make you more comfortable while gardening. A hat with a wide brim helps keep you cool and protects the eyes and face from strong sunlight. Sunglasses and sunscreen are good to keep in your kit for gardening, too. Also take a bottle of water with you when you head outside so you can stay hydrated and comfortable.

To avoid injury and discomfort, don't hunch over, keep your back straight while you work, and avoid twisting. Instead of bending or kneeling, try squatting down. It is actually an easier way to work. It may feel awkward at first but it is good for the hips and an antidote for sitting too much. Lift using the power of your legs by bending your knees instead of relying on your back muscles. Gardening is good exercise as long as we do it mindfully.

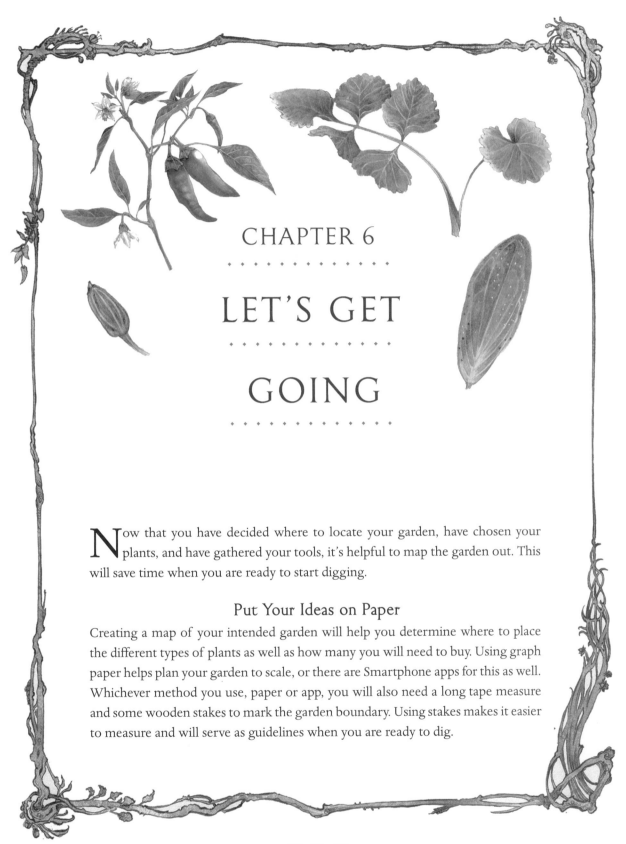

CHAPTER 6

· · · · · · · · ·

LET'S GET

· · · · · · · · ·

GOING

· · · · · · · · ·

Now that you have decided where to locate your garden, have chosen your plants, and have gathered your tools, it's helpful to map the garden out. This will save time when you are ready to start digging.

Put Your Ideas on Paper

Creating a map of your intended garden will help you determine where to place the different types of plants as well as how many you will need to buy. Using graph paper helps plan your garden to scale, or there are Smartphone apps for this as well. Whichever method you use, paper or app, you will also need a long tape measure and some wooden stakes to mark the garden boundary. Using stakes makes it easier to measure and will serve as guidelines when you are ready to dig.

Once you measure the outline of the garden, sketch in adjacent features such as shrubs, a wall, or a patio. If you have a big old tree like I do, you may need to note where some of its large roots extend above ground. Include paths, stepping stones, or any other feature you may be thinking of adding to the space. After the "hard" features are on paper, you are ready to sketch the plants. These can be indicated as circles for the areas each type of plant will occupy or a circle for each individual plant. Your map can be as detailed or as broadly defined as you prefer. Whenever possible, plant the same type of herb in groups of three for a cohesive appearance rather than scattering them all over. A small grouping is visually pleasing but does not present a large target for pests to zero in on.

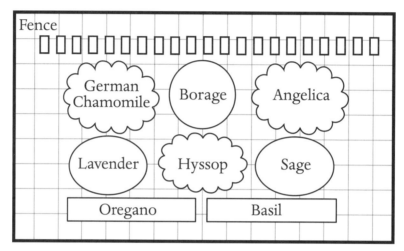

Figure 1.4. A garden layout on paper can be simple or detailed and is a time-saver when you are ready to plant.

While you have paper handy, you may want to consider keeping a garden journal. This way you will know what you planted each year and you will have a record of what worked well and what did not. There are ready-made gardening journals, but making your own and adding pictures or seed packets or even pressing a few leaves or flowers inside can be an interesting and fun way to track the progress of your garden from year to year. In addition, keeping track of how you dealt with pests and the results of your harvests can provide valuable information in the years ahead. Your journal can be as simple or elaborate as you care to make it. The important thing is that it be fun and interesting for you.

How to Lay Out Your Plan

The first step in starting a new garden is to establish its outer edges. Mark the corners with stakes and use string to define the outline. If your design calls for flowing instead of straight borders, use more stakes and a garden hose or a rope to define the boundary. For a round garden, put a stake in what will be the center and attach a piece of string that is a little longer than the garden's radius (half its diameter). Fill a bottle with sand and then attach it to the other end of the string, making it the length of the radius. Slowly walk in a circle shaking out a little sand as you go to define the outer boundary of the garden.

Once you have defined the outer edges of your garden, step back and take a look to make sure it is the size and shape you want. You can always expand a garden later but if it seems too big, now is the time to adjust your plan. If you are including paths in your garden, also mark these with stakes and string.

When first digging a garden, begin at the outer edges to establish the border. If you are starting with bare ground, remove any fallen branches, rocks, or other debris and then turn over the soil with a shovel or a spading fork. Over time, soil packs together and loosening it allows roots to grow more easily. This will also help water to penetrate the soil as well as drain away.

If you are claiming a piece of lawn for a garden, you will need to get rid of the grass. There are several ways to do this. In the autumn, put down a thick layer of mulch or cover the area with a couple of inches of newspaper, and then cover it with a thin layer of topsoil. The grass will die back and the newspaper will disintegrate. Instead of waiting for mulch or newspaper to smother the grass or if you are starting in the spring, you can simply turn the grass under. Break up each shovelful of soil and pull out big clumps of grass and roots to prevent them from getting reestablished.

While the ground may look level, once you start working it you may find a lot of bumps and dips. In addition to dealing with these, you may find that one end is higher than the other. If so, find a medium point and redistribute the soil with a rake to make it as level as you can. If paving stones or bricks are part of your plan, dig out those areas, too, even if you are placing a few stepping stones here and there. Digging out the path will make it easier to create a stable base so the stones won't become uneven as they settle. Another reason to dig out the entire garden area is to rid it of any bindweed or knotweed roots that creep underground and make their presence known where you least expect them. I'm sure my neighbors thought I was a real crackpot doing so much digging when I was starting my garden, but I was battling Japanese knotweed, and my vigilance paid off.

When laying out a path, dig to double the depth of the bricks or stones. Tamp down the ground and then put in a thick layer of gravel and sand. This will create a stable base on which to set the stones. Consider leaving a little space between the stones or bricks where low-growing herbs such as creeping thyme or Roman chamomile can grow.

After the paths or stepping stones are in place, continue to dig out the remaining bedding areas. If your garden is bordered by a lawn, adding a hard edge helps keep the grass from creeping in. A wide range of ready-made edging material is available at garden centers or you can use bricks or stones. Dig down a little to sink part of each border stone or brick into the ground so they will stay in place.

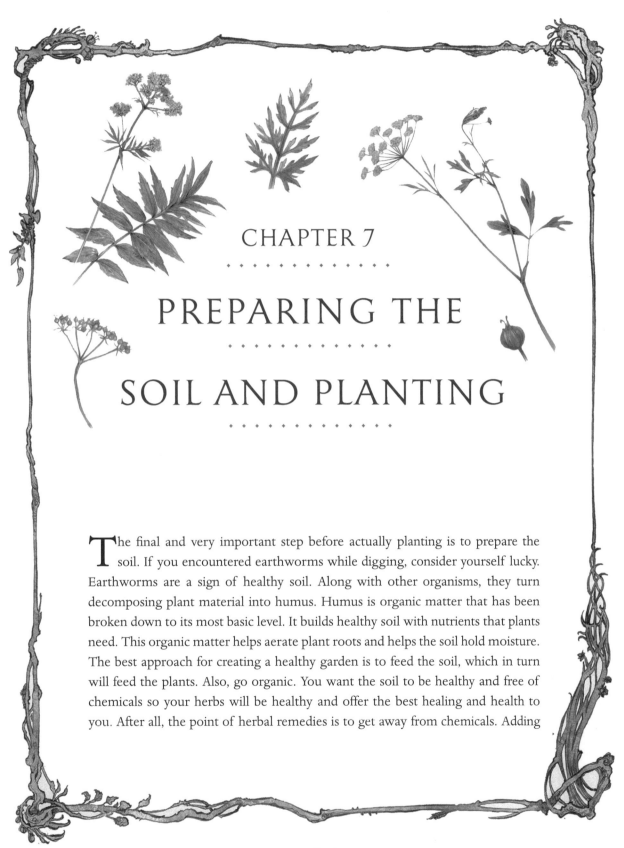

CHAPTER 7

· · · · · · · · · · · · · · · · · ·

PREPARING THE

· · · · · · · · · · · · · · · · · ·

SOIL AND PLANTING

· · · · · · · · · · · · · · · · · ·

The final and very important step before actually planting is to prepare the soil. If you encountered earthworms while digging, consider yourself lucky. Earthworms are a sign of healthy soil. Along with other organisms, they turn decomposing plant material into humus. Humus is organic matter that has been broken down to its most basic level. It builds healthy soil with nutrients that plants need. This organic matter helps aerate plant roots and helps the soil hold moisture. The best approach for creating a healthy garden is to feed the soil, which in turn will feed the plants. Also, go organic. You want the soil to be healthy and free of chemicals so your herbs will be healthy and offer the best healing and health to you. After all, the point of herbal remedies is to get away from chemicals. Adding chemicals to the soil means that you are adding them to your herbs, which in turn gets ingested by you and your family.

Fertilizer, Compost, and Mulch: Wondering What to Use?

A stroll through a garden center may give you the impression that you will need to put a lot of different stuff on your garden. Truth be told, you don't. Building and maintaining healthy soil is not complicated or difficult, and it does not require you to buy a lot of bags of different stuff.

The first thing that comes to mind, of course, is to use fertilizer for a healthy garden. The problem is, many fertilizers are synthetic, and, while they may produce bigger plants, they do not enrich the soil. They do not feed the earthworms and microorganisms that build healthy soil. Plants may get a good initial boost from fertilizer, but the state of the soil will decline and then the plants will too. To save the plants you then have to add more fertilizer. The result is that your garden will be thrown into the vicious cycle of feast or famine. To avoid this, use an organic fertilizer that will not cause this problem because it feeds the plants while it also builds healthy soil.

Before saying "fertilizer, yuck," you may be thinking that organic fertilizer means manure, but there is a big difference. While manure may be used as fertilizer, fertilizer doesn't have to include manure. Manure is animal waste, and pets should never be considered as a source for manure. The waste from cats and dogs not only smells bad but it contains harmful bacteria that can make people sick. It can also harbor parasites. Fresh manure from barnyard animals is equally bad. Any urine that was mixed in with the manure has a burning effect on herbs. Then there's E. coli, salmonella, and other problems. Bagged manure that has been processed to kill E. coli and other pathogens is available at some garden centers. However, if it isn't guaranteed to have come from an organic farm, there is the risk of pesticide residues, antibiotics, and other medications that may have been given to the livestock. In my opinion, it is not worth the risk.

The best thing you can use on your garden is compost. Compost is a natural fertilizer that conditions the soil, improving drainage as well as the capacity to retain water. Compost speeds up the process of organic breakdown, keeping the earthworms and microorganisms happy, which in turn produces healthy plants. The best thing of all, it's free because we can make it ourselves. There are special compost bins on the market, but it's not necessary to use them or any bin for that matter. I keep a good, old-fashioned compost pile. The advantage to using a bin is that it keeps the temperature of the material hotter, which speeds up the process. Whichever method you use, the important thing to remember is that compost needs to be turned a couple of times a month otherwise it will disintegrate into a useless, slimy mess.

A compost pile can be unsightly, but it is easily hidden by creating a small fenced-in area that is open on one side for easy access. Because the pile should not rest against wood, as the wood will rot over time, it works well to stack a few cinder blocks to create an enclosure and then surround the blocks with a decorative fence or shrubs. Locate your compost pile on level ground where it won't get direct sunlight and where it will have good drainage.

Compost is made with soil, vegetable and fruit scraps, leaves, small twigs, grass clippings, straw, shredded newspaper, coffee grounds, used tea leaves, and plant trimmings. At the end of the summer, I empty the contents of my flower boxes onto the pile, too. Also, instead of throwing out plant material after making infusions or other remedies, add them to your compost pile. Avoid cooked fruit and veggie scraps, meat, and milk products, as these cause odors and attract rats.

Start the pile on bare ground with a couple of inches of small twigs. This aids in getting air into the pile to help start the process. Shovel a couple of inches of soil over the twigs and then add the organic material listed above. Try to use a mix of things; not just vegetable scraps or not just grass clippings. Top off the pile with a thin layer of soil. Wet it down, but don't make it soggy. Use a shovel to turn the pile over a few times a month especially when you add new material. Moisten the pile each time. Turning the pile helps to aerate the material, which aids the process of decomposition. The compost will be ready to use in a few months when it becomes dark and crumbly. Shovel the compost on top of the soil in the your garden, use a rake to mix it in, and then water.

If you are growing chamomile, add spent flower heads after making remedies or any part of the plant to the compost pile as it is a good activator to get the process going. Yarrow is also a good activator. Another very beneficial item to add to your compost pile is seaweed. Even if you are not near the coast, seaweed in liquid and powder form is available at some garden centers. Using seaweed in the garden is beneficial because it adds trace minerals to the soil. If you are near a beach, go at low tide to gather a few handfuls of seaweed. Dry it, crumble it up, and mix it into your compost.

Last but not least, there's mulch. The first thing to know about mulch is that there are two varieties: organic and inorganic. In this case, "organic" does not refer to it being free from pesticides, it means that it came from something that was living at one time. This type of mulch is made of wood chips, shredded bark, straw, leaves, grass clippings, pine needles, sawdust, or paper. An organic mulch will break down and feed the soil. If you decide to use mulch, look for an organic mulch that came from a pesticide-free source. Cocoa shells are also used for mulch, however, while they smell nice (who doesn't like a chocolaty aroma?), they are toxic to cats and dogs. The inorganic mulches are made of gravel or plastic and, obviously, will not enrich the soil.

The purpose of mulch is to hold in moisture and regulate the temperature of the soil. It keeps plants cool in the summer and protects them in the winter. In addition, mulch helps deter weeds and pests. However, instead of buying mulch, you can use grass clippings, leaves, or compost. As previously mentioned, compost is worked into the soil, however, when it is used as a mulch, it is left on top of the soil and not raked in.

When using any type of mulch, dampen the ground, pull out weeds, and then layer the mulch about an inch deep around the plants. Be sure to leave some space around the stems so air can circulate, which will prevent rot. Mulch after plants are at least six inches tall so they won't be buried and it will be easier to get the mulch underneath them. Slugs and snails really like mulch, so try to leave about eight inches of bare ground around the mulch. Grass clippings make a good mulch for annuals as they release a lot of nitrogen that these plants need. While mulch is applied in deeper layers to other types of gardens, it can keep the soil too moist for most herbs, which can encourage the growth of fungus. Be sure to follow the needs for your particular plants.

Planting Your Herbs

If you are new to gardening, buying plants the first season will serve as a good introduction for the tasks involved. Make a list of the plants that you want (common and scientific names) and take it with you to the garden center. Look for plants that seem sturdy and have short spaces between the leaves rather than ones that are tall and leggy. Also, look for ones that have a healthy color and are free from pests.

At some point, if you decide to try your hand at starting herbs from seed, sow them indoors about three months before the growing season in your area. Seed packets should have both the common and scientific names for the plant as well as planting instructions. Also, check the packet to make sure the seeds were not treated with chemicals.

Items needed for starting your herbs from seed include seed trays that are divided into sections, a bag of potting mix, and a spray bottle. Consider recycling plastic egg cartons for seed trays. Other alternatives to seed trays are peat or newspaper pots, which are biodegradable and can be planted directly in the ground, where they will decompose. A potting soil mix or a seed starter mix are blends of mediums that aid seed germination. A spray bottle is good to use because the seeds need to be kept moist, but we don't want to drown them.

Whether you are sowing seeds indoors or outside when it's warmer, start the day before by soaking the seeds in warm water overnight, which will help them to germinate. When you are ready to sow, place a little potting mix in the seed tray, drop in several seeds per compartment or pot, cover with soil, and use the spray bottle to gently water. Most seed trays come with lids, and if you are using the clear plastic egg crates, they have built-in lids. Otherwise, use a piece of plastic wrap and make a tent over your seed pots. Covering them helps to create a warm, moist atmosphere. Place them in a warm, dark spot, which will aid the germination process. Check them every day for sprouts.

When seedlings begin to appear, remove the lid or tent, and keep them in a warm, bright spot out of direct sunlight, which is too harsh for these baby plants. If there are multiple seedlings per compartment, remove some of them and leave only the strongest one or two. After the seedlings develop several sets of leaves, transplant them into separate small pots so the roots will have room to develop. Put soil in the pot and make a well in the middle. Remove a seedling from the tray with a teaspoon and carefully place it in the pot. Gently fill in soil around the roots. Continue to keep the plants moist but not wet. If you are using the biodegradable peat or newspaper pots, you will not have to repot the seedlings. Let the plants develop for a few weeks.

Whether you purchase plants or start them from seed, they need to go through a process called "hardening off," which takes a few days. After all threat of frost has passed, move the plants outdoors in stages so they can gradually adjust to the light and temperature in your garden. Move the pots out to a porch or sheltered area for a day or two, and then place them in the garden where you will plant them for another day or two. Plant them in the ground on a cloudy day or after three in the afternoon so they will not be in the direct, hot sunlight right away.

Using your trowel, dig a hole for each plant. Follow the needs of your plants for spacing to avoid overcrowding. Plants release moisture from their leaves and when they are too close together the humidity level around them is elevated, which can foster the growth of bacteria and fungus. Crowded plants have to compete for resources of soil and sun and do not get as strong and well developed as those that don't struggle to survive. To remove a plant from its pot, water it, gently tilt the pot, and then carefully slide it out. Support the plant as you fill soil in around the roots and pat it gently but don't pack it down. When all the plants are in the ground, give them a good watering.

Seeds can also be started directly outside. Unlike those sown indoors, you can't get a jump on the season because the ground must be warm enough. Follow the information on the seed packets. When you are ready to sow, make one-inch diameter holes in the soil and drop in two or three seeds per hole. Cover with soil and pat lightly. To make sure that you remember where everything is, mark each area with the name of the herb using special tags available at garden centers, or use Popsicle sticks. For a unique look, write the herb names on wine corks, poke each cork onto one end of a wooden barbecue skewer, and stick the other end of the skewer in the ground. Keep the soil moist until seedlings sprout. Thin them by pulling out extras so they are at the distance indicated on the seed packet to avoid overcrowding.

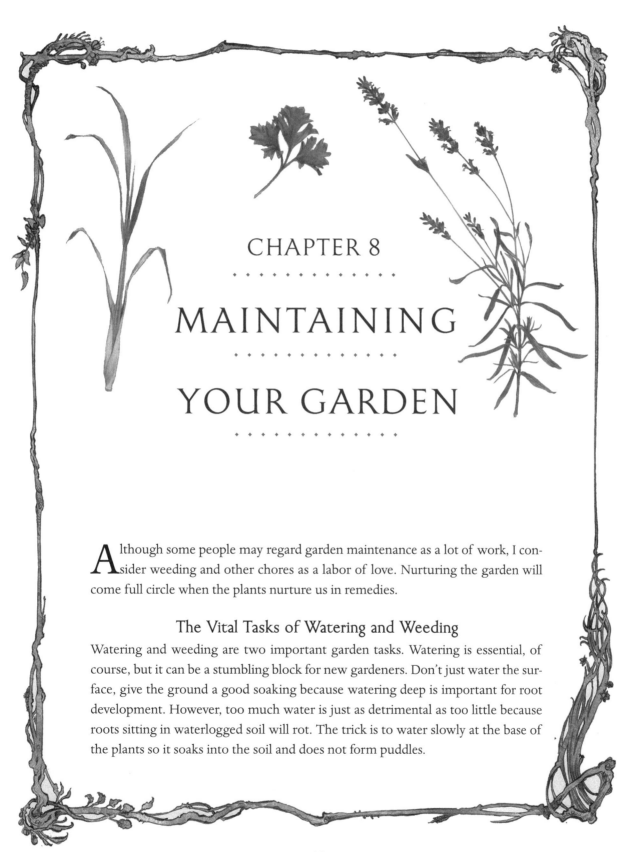

CHAPTER 8

· · · · · · · · ·

MAINTAINING

· · · · · · · · ·

YOUR GARDEN

· · · · · · · · ·

Although some people may regard garden maintenance as a lot of work, I consider weeding and other chores as a labor of love. Nurturing the garden will come full circle when the plants nurture us in remedies.

The Vital Tasks of Watering and Weeding

Watering and weeding are two important garden tasks. Watering is essential, of course, but it can be a stumbling block for new gardeners. Don't just water the surface, give the ground a good soaking because watering deep is important for root development. However, too much water is just as detrimental as too little because roots sitting in waterlogged soil will rot. The trick is to water slowly at the base of the plants so it soaks into the soil and does not form puddles.

Because temperatures and humidity are constantly changing, when and how much you water will vary throughout the season. Use your fingers to check for moisture a couple of inches below the surface of the soil, and then follow the needs for the types of herbs you have planted. By paying attention to how quickly or slowly the soil dries out, you will get a good feel for the particular needs of your garden. Water the garden early in the morning. This way, the water will soak into the soil rather than evaporate during the heat of the day. Watering early also gives the foliage time to dry, which helps avoid the development of fungal disease.

Plan to spend some time each week removing weeds. Most herbs are slow growers and weeds can quickly take over, robbing them of water resources and space. The greatest amount of weeds show up in the early part of the season, so keeping them under control is important when herbs are in the early stages of their growth cycle and just getting established. As previously mentioned, mulch helps keep weeds down but too much can keep the soil too moist for many herbs. It may seem like a fine line to walk, but experiment to see whether mulching or not mulching works best for your garden.

Be sure to get rid of weeds before they go to seed or you will have a lot more to contend with later. Pull them out by hand and dig as little as possible to avoid disturbing herb roots. Also, weeding is easier after a rain shower when the ground is soft. Doing a little weeding often is an easy way to keep them in check.

Propagation: Making More Plants

At some point you may want to propagate your plants so you have more without having to purchase them. There are four methods that are easy to do, however, not all plants can be propagated by all four methods. Specific information on appropriate propagation methods is included for each herb in part 3. The four propagation methods are seed, division, cutting, and layering.

Seed: Starting plants from seed was covered in the previous chapter. Seeds can be purchased or you can gather them from many of your existing plants.

Division: This refers to dividing the plant's roots. To do this, dig up the entire root ball and then pull it apart into two or three pieces. Some fibrous roots may need to be cut apart. While this can be done with a shovel, a spading fork makes this task easier. Once the root ball has been separated, dig a hole for each piece and plant them. This can be done in the autumn, however, if you do it in the spring the new plants will have more time to get established.

Cutting: Starting at the top of the plant, move down at least five leaves and cut off the top part of a stem. Cut on an angle rather than straight across to expose more of the interior stem. Remove a few of the bottom leaves from the cutting to have enough of a stem to plant. Place it in a container with potting mix and set it away from direct sunlight. Keep the soil moist, but not soggy. The cutting will produce its own root system.

Layering: In this method, a piece of stem produces its own root system before being cut from the original plant. Carefully bend a lower stem so part of it lays along the ground. It helps to pin it in place. To make some pins, take a wire coat hanger and cut the sides off creating a U-shaped wire. Carefully push one pin into the ground to gently hold the stem in place. If necessary, use two pins. Cover that part of the stem with a little soil and water it. That is the point at which it will develop roots. Give it a few weeks and then carefully move some of the soil to check for roots. If they have developed, cut the stem close to the original plant and transplant the new one in its own location.

Winter Care: Tuck Your Garden in for the Season

At least several weeks before frost is expected, turn under the soil where any annuals grew and cut back the other herbs. If you have a fireplace, keep woody stems of lavender to toss into the fire during the winter for an aromatic treat. Autumn leaves are timed perfectly for use as a protective winter mulch around the base of biennials and perennials. Mulching will also prevent erosion from rain and snow melt. Straw also makes a good winter mulch.

An easy way to mulch is to scatter oat seeds around the garden and cover lightly with soil. In a week or two little shoots will appear. Don't worry about oats overtaking the garden because the first good frost will kill it off. The grassy oat leaves create a mulch that can be turned over and worked into the soil in the spring. No matter what you use as mulch, in the early spring after the threat of frost ends pull the mulch back from the base of the plants to allow air circulation around the stems, which will prevent rot.

Depending on your zone, tender perennials may need to be over-wintered in a garage or in the house. If the herbs were not grown in containers, transplant them into pots. Just like hardening off in the spring, gradually move the potted herbs to their new locations so they have time to adjust to the different conditions. Also, check that you are not moving pests inside, which could infest other houseplants. Make sure these new indoor plants get the right amount of sunlight.

After the harvest and clean up, the remaining parts of plants can go on the compost pile. Like the garden, tucking your compost pile in for the season will protect it. Some microbes remain active in the winter and protecting the pile will have it ready to go earlier next spring. If you created the pile with cinder blocks, bricks, or stones, your protective barrier is already in place. Securing a tarp over it can help keep it dry. Another way to get it ready for winter is to put leaves and branches on the compost pile and then top it off with some soil. After the winter holidays, I recycle my Yule wreath by placing it on top of the pile. This works nicely to protect it and in the spring I chop the wreath into small pieces and mix them in with the compost.

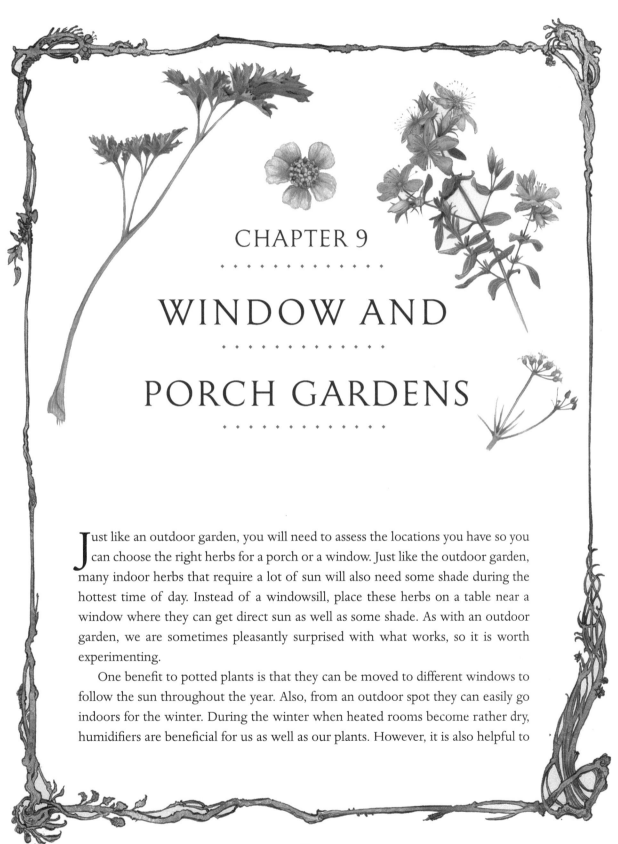

CHAPTER 9

• • • • • • •

WINDOW AND

• • • • • • • •

PORCH GARDENS

• • • • • • • • •

Just like an outdoor garden, you will need to assess the locations you have so you can choose the right herbs for a porch or a window. Just like the outdoor garden, many indoor herbs that require a lot of sun will also need some shade during the hottest time of day. Instead of a windowsill, place these herbs on a table near a window where they can get direct sun as well as some shade. As with an outdoor garden, we are sometimes pleasantly surprised with what works, so it is worth experimenting.

One benefit to potted plants is that they can be moved to different windows to follow the sun throughout the year. Also, from an outdoor spot they can easily go indoors for the winter. During the winter when heated rooms become rather dry, humidifiers are beneficial for us as well as our plants. However, it is also helpful to occasionally spray the leaves with tepid water to give them a boost. Avoid windowsills that are just above radiators as plants will dry out quickly and not do well with the fluctuating temperatures.

Don't feel constrained by conventional flowerpots. Containers for plants can be varied and imaginative. A neighbor of mine used several old metal coffee pots as planters. Anything can be used as long as it provides good drainage, which means you may have to drill a hole or two into something that did not start its life as a flowerpot. An old basket can be recycled to hold a collection of small flowerpots.

Several types of herbs can be grouped together in one pot and pots can be arranged together to create an interesting display. Just like an outdoor garden, position a tall plant in the center of a flowerpot with shorter ones around it. As mentioned in chapter 3, peppermint and spearmint have rambunctious root systems that tend to take over the garden. The easiest way to deal with this is to grow them in containers even if you have an outdoor garden. They should be given containers of their own because they will crowd out any other plant that may be sharing the flowerpot with them. Here are some herbs that do well when grown in containers:

- Basil
- Bay
- Cayenne
- Chamomile
- Dill
- Garlic
- Lavender
- Lemon balm
- Lemongrass
- Marjoram
- Parsley
- Peppermint*
- Sage
- Spearmint*
- Thyme
- Yarrow

*These plants should be in a container by themselves.

When planting in containers, use ones that are large enough to allow room for the roots to grow. If the container is too small, plants become root-bound, which means the roots will fill the pot and the plants will do poorly. Start with a layer of gravel or seashells, which will help provide drainage and keep the bottom part of the soil from becoming waterlogged. Also, if you are growing perennials, you will need to repot them into larger containers as they grow.

Good soil is key for any type of garden. When growing plants in containers, use potting mix rather than potting soil. Bagged potting soil is often too thick and clumpy and will result in poor drainage. A potting mix includes peat or composted plant matter and gives container plants the texture and drainage they need.

Plants in containers have a smaller amount of soil from which to draw nutrients, so it is important to add a little compost during the growing season. Instead of compost, you can use a "compost tea." To make the tea you will need a bucket and a muslin or cotton bag large enough to hold several handfuls of compost. Once you fill the bag, tie it closed, put it in the bucket, and fill it with water. Let it soak for three days, return the compost to the pile, and use the tea to water your plants.

Hanging baskets and flower boxes work well on porches where space may be at a premium. If a porch or balcony gets a lot of wind, secure a small trellis to a railing to act as a windbreak. On a balcony, you may want to use lightweight pots instead of clay ones to avoid adding too much weight to the structure. Even if you have an outdoor garden, consider using a few potted herbs to provide a focal point and variety.

While I have some herbs scattered around my flower gardens, I grow most of them in containers on my back porch. The sunlight is just right there and I can easily move them indoors to a table by my sunny kitchen window.

Part 2 provides details on how to harvest and prepare herbs for storage. It also contains information on how to make and use herbal preparations as well as information on essential and carrier oils.

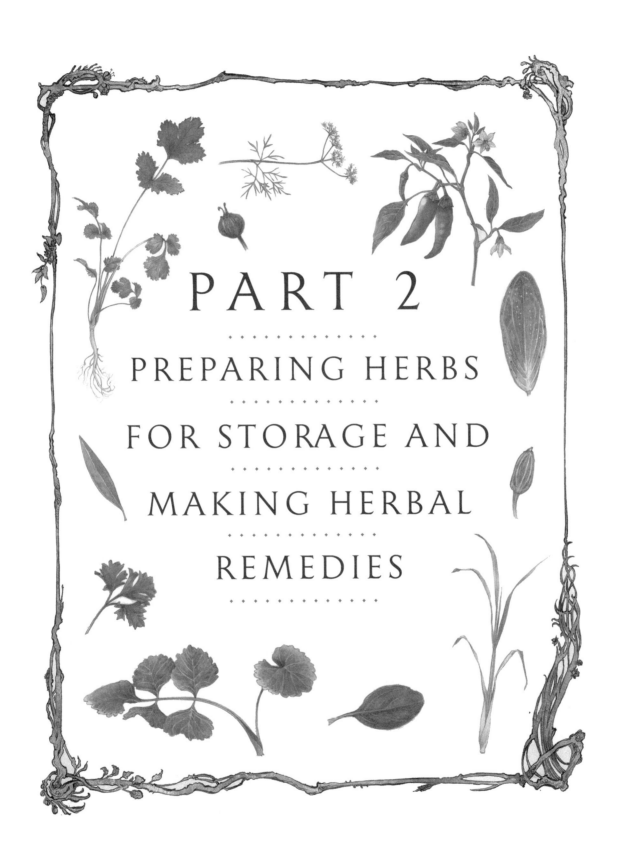

PART 2

· · · · · · · · · · · · · ·

PREPARING HERBS

· · · · · · · · · · · · · ·

FOR STORAGE AND

· · · · · · · · · · · · · ·

MAKING HERBAL

· · · · · · · · · · · · · ·

REMEDIES

· · · · · · · · · · · · · ·

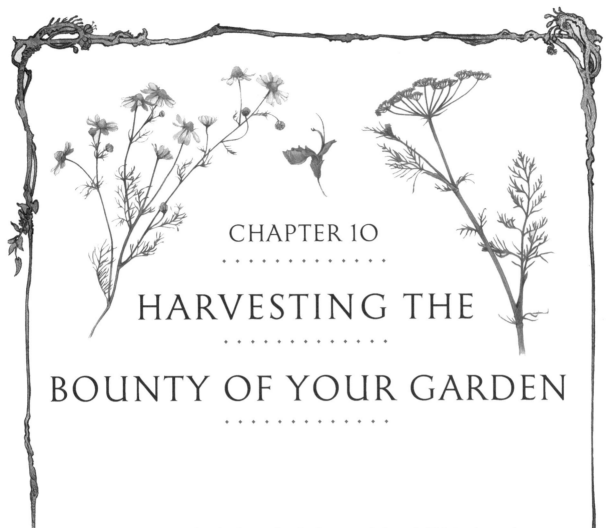

CHAPTER 10

· · · · · · · ·

HARVESTING THE

· · · · · · · · · · ·

BOUNTY OF YOUR GARDEN

· · · · · · · · · · · · · ·

Harvesting needs to be done when herbs are at their peak. This is when a plant is at its most vital and will yield the best flavor, fragrance, and healing properties. Here are some general guidelines for when to harvest various parts of plants:

Flowers	The day they open or just before fully opened
Leaves	Before the flowers bloom
Seeds	When they are ripe
Roots	*Annuals:* Anytime in the season when the plant has finished its life cycle *Biennials:* The autumn of their first year or the following spring *Perennials:* Fall, winter, or spring

The tools needed for harvesting include pruning shears, scissors, shovel, trowel, and a couple of baskets or buckets. Harvest leaves and flowers on a dry day just after the dew evaporates. Do not gather plants that show signs of insect damage, mildew, or any disease. If you plan to use herbs fresh, store them in a sealed plastic bag or a container in the fridge. Leaves and flowers can be kept a day or two this way before use. Do not rinse them off before storing because they will not keep well. Gardening organic means that we don't need to worry about cleaning off pesticides. Also, washing after picking may cause the loss of some essential oil, which is important for many healing properties.

Flowers can be harvested by hand or with scissors. Handle them gently to avoid bruising. Don't harvest flowers that look like they are fading, as they will be past their peak. Dirty ones cannot be washed and dried successfully so it is best to put those directly on the compost pile. Use scissors to harvest stems and leaves. Do not pull leaves off as this may damage the plant. Brush or shake off any dirt or bugs.

Herbs grown for their leaves are usually harvested throughout the season and before the plants flower. Leaves often become coarse and lose their flavor after the plant blooms. After harvesting mints, lemon balm, and marjoram in the summer, the plants can be pruned down to the first set of leaves. Don't worry, you're not killing the plants, they will spring back with new growth and give you a second harvest. Basil and parsley can also be cut back throughout the season to encourage new growth.

Seeds usually start out green and then turn a different color when ripe. They can be left to ripen on the plant before harvesting, but keep an eye on them by checking each day because the seeds will drop to the ground. You will need a cloth or a paper bag to harvest them. When they appear to be ripe, gently bend the stalk until the seed head is over a cloth placed on the ground or inside a paper bag. Shake the plant so the seeds fall onto the cloth or into the bag. Alternatively, once the seed head is in a bag, cut the stalk off the plant. Poke holes in the bag for air circulation, hang it somewhere dry, and just let the seeds fall off when they are ready.

Roots should be harvested in the autumn or early spring when the plant's energy is in its roots, making them more potent. Of course, if you are going to harvest the leaves or other parts of these plants do so first, then harvest the roots. On a day when the soil is moist, not wet, use a shovel, spading fork, or trowel (depending on the size of the plant) to loosen the ground around it. Get the shovel under the roots and gently pry the whole plant from the soil. Trim off stems to within one inch of the root and wipe off any excess soil.

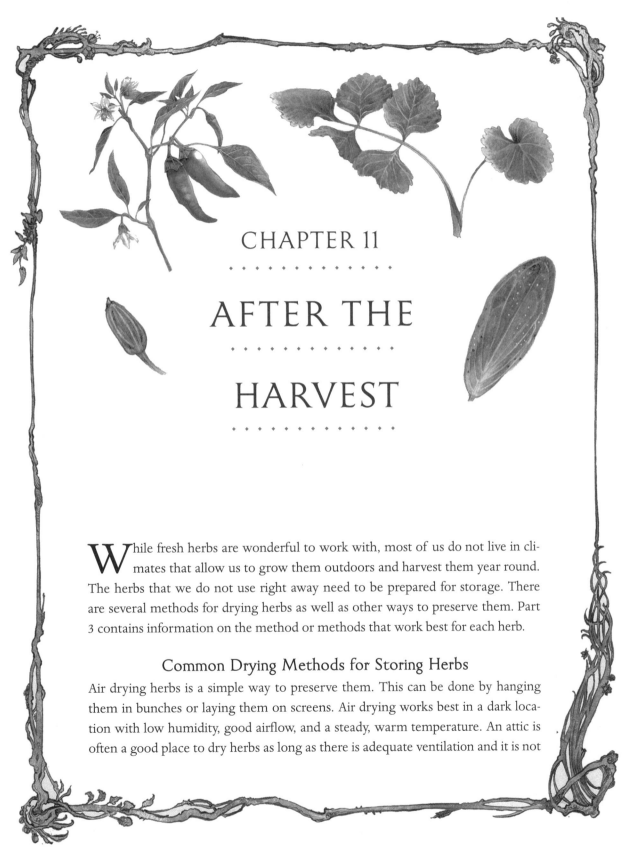

CHAPTER 11

· · · · · · · · ·

AFTER THE

· · · · · · · · ·

HARVEST

· · · · · · · · ·

While fresh herbs are wonderful to work with, most of us do not live in climates that allow us to grow them outdoors and harvest them year round. The herbs that we do not use right away need to be prepared for storage. There are several methods for drying herbs as well as other ways to preserve them. Part 3 contains information on the method or methods that work best for each herb.

Common Drying Methods for Storing Herbs

Air drying herbs is a simple way to preserve them. This can be done by hanging them in bunches or laying them on screens. Air drying works best in a dark location with low humidity, good airflow, and a steady, warm temperature. An attic is often a good place to dry herbs as long as there is adequate ventilation and it is not excessively dusty. However, you may need to block some of the light from any window to darken the drying area. It does not need to be pitch black; just avoid bright sunlight. You may find the right conditions in a corner of a room, a porch, a shed, or even a large closet where linens or clothes can be scented as the herbs dry. Whatever spot you choose, air circulation is a key factor.

Gather herbs early in the day and do not rinse them unless they are muddy. If you do rinse them, lay the herbs out on paper towels and let them dry before gathering into bunches. It is important to bundle the same type of herb together rather than mixing them because different plants dry at different rates. Basil, borage, lemon balm, and mints have high moisture contents and dry more slowly than sage, rosemary, and thyme.

Tie up to ten stems into bundles. Herbs that take longer to dry should be tied into smaller bundles of about five or less. Fasten the bunches together with rubber bands, twist ties, or yarn. Attach several bunches, upside down, to a wire coat hanger with enough space between them so air can circulate freely. A wooden laundry rack can be set up wherever the conditions are right and can hold a number of herb-ladened coat hangers. If you don't have a lot of herbs to dry, the bunches can be attached directly to the laundry rack. Whichever way you hang the herbs, make sure the bunches are not touching each other and that they are not right up against a wall or other structure. If you are concerned about dust, tie cheesecloth around each bunch or drape it over the whole laundry rack if you are using one.

For screen drying herbs, a clean window screen works well. As an alternative, a piece of cheesecloth, muslin, or brown paper with small holes poked through it can be attached to an old picture frame to make a drying screen. Whatever you use for a screen, lay out the herbs in a single layer. The screens can be set on laundry racks, which will allow good air circulation. The leaves of bay, peppermint, spearmint, and sage dry better when they are removed from the stems and screen dried.

Check your screens and bundles every day and take herbs down as soon as they are dry. They will feel slightly brittle when they are completely dry. Store the herbs immediately, otherwise they will start to deteriorate. If you hung herbs in bundles, strip the leaves and/or flowers from the stems for storage. Use glass jars with tight lids, and avoid metal containers as they can taint the herbs. Store the jars in a cool place away from sunlight. Dried herbs can keep for up to a year or a little longer. If you notice a mist or moisture inside a jar, take the herbs out and dry them a little longer.

For seeds, the harvest can continue indoors. As mentioned in chapter 10, seed heads can be hung upside down in a paper bag, which will catch the seeds as they fall. Poke holes in the sides of the bag for air circulation. It may take a week or two for the seeds to drop. After this, they can be dried. Some seeds may be inside a husk or a shell, which will have to be removed. Gently pry the husk or shell open. Chaff, which are pieces of husk or shell that may stick to the seeds, can be wiped off. Place the seeds in a glass jar with a piece of cheesecloth fastened over the opening. It can take from three to ten days for them to completely dry. Reshuffling the seeds helps them to dry, so each day transfer the seeds into another jar. After four or five days, test the dryness by pressing your fingernail into one of the seeds. If it is hard, the seeds are dry. Transfer them a final time into a clean jar with a tight lid for storage. If the test seed was somewhat soft, continue moving them back and forth into different jars for a few more days.

If you are keeping seeds for planting a new crop of herbs, put them in an envelope and mark it with the name of the plant and when the seeds were harvested. Put the envelope in a freezer storage bag or a container and then put it in the freezer. Most seeds will be viable for three to seven years.

After roots are harvested, wash and scrub them with water, and then cut them into small, one- or two-inch pieces for drying. The cut roots can be kept in the fridge up to forty-eight hours before drying. Because they are dense, roots take longer to dry than other parts of plants. However, the process can be jump-started by using the oven. Place a layer of paper towels on a cookie sheet and spread out the root pieces. Set the oven at the lowest temperature for three to four hours. Leave the door open slightly to allow air circulation and to keep the roots from baking. Check them every hour and turn them over for uniform drying. Transfer the roots to a screen and place it in a warm room to complete the drying process.

Using the oven is a quicker way to dry leaves and flowers, however, some of the essential oils will be lost, which means some flavor and potency are, too. If you opt for this method, follow the same instructions as for drying roots. Leaves and flowers may take two to four hours to dry. When they are crisp, remove them from the oven. Allow them to cool thoroughly before storing.

The microwave can also be used to remove moisture from herbs. Lay them out in a single layer between two paper towels. Microwave them for a minute at a time. It may take about four minutes for them to dry, but this way you can check their progress and turn them over so they dry evenly. Replace the paper towels when they get moist. Stop microwaving the herbs when they are crisp, and allow them to cool before storing.

Dehydrators can also be used to dry herbs. Line the trays with cheesecloth to keep small flowers and leaves from falling through to lower trays. Set the temperature between 90° and 100° Fahrenheit. Leaves and flowers may take a day or two, and roots three days or more.

Freezing and Other Methods for Storage

Freezing is the easiest method for preserving herbs. It works especially well for basil, cilantro, dill, fennel, lemongrass, mint, parsley, and thyme. Some herbs, such as basil, may lose color and texture, but they retain their flavor and potency. To prepare herbs for freezing, lay them out in a single layer on a baking sheet and place it in the freezer. Once the herbs are frozen, store them in freezer bags or plastic containers. Herbs can be frozen whole or they can be chopped up first.

Put some chopped peppermint in an ice cube tray and add a little water. These can be used to flavor drinks, or you can drop a couple of ice cubes into a mug and pour in boiling water for tea. Also, herbs can be pureed in a food processor with a little water and then frozen in ice cube trays. Once they set, remove the cubes from the trays and store them in bags or containers. These are ready to go when you want to make a tea, infusion, or other preparation. If there are certain combinations of herbs that you enjoy using, puree them together and freeze. Also consider pureeing herbs with a little olive oil. Basil and cilantro work well this way.

Another way to preserve leaves is to dry them with non-iodized table salt or sea salt. Place a layer of salt in a shallow pan, lay the leaves on the salt, and then sprinkle enough salt over top to completely cover them. It usually takes two to four weeks for leaves to dry with this method. Check from time to time by digging out a leaf. Rebury it if necessary. When they are dry, dig them out of the salt and shake off any excess. Store the leaves in glass jars in a cupboard away from light. Rinse them in cold water before using to remove any remaining salt.

Strong-flavored herbs can be preserved in oil, vinegar, or brandy. Basil mixed with sea salt and covered with olive oil can last several years. Although the leaves will blacken, the flavor and potency remain intact. Mint is often preserved in white, red, or wine vinegar. Mint can also be preserved with olive oil. To steep in brandy, fill a jar with the herb, add brandy, and store tightly covered for a month. The herb material can be strained out or left in. Small quantities of the brandy can be used as a cordial or, depending on the herb, as a digestive aid.

Now that you have harvested and stored your herbs, they will be handy and ready when you need to prepare remedies. But first, let's learn about essential and carrier oils so we can incorporate them into our healing remedies.

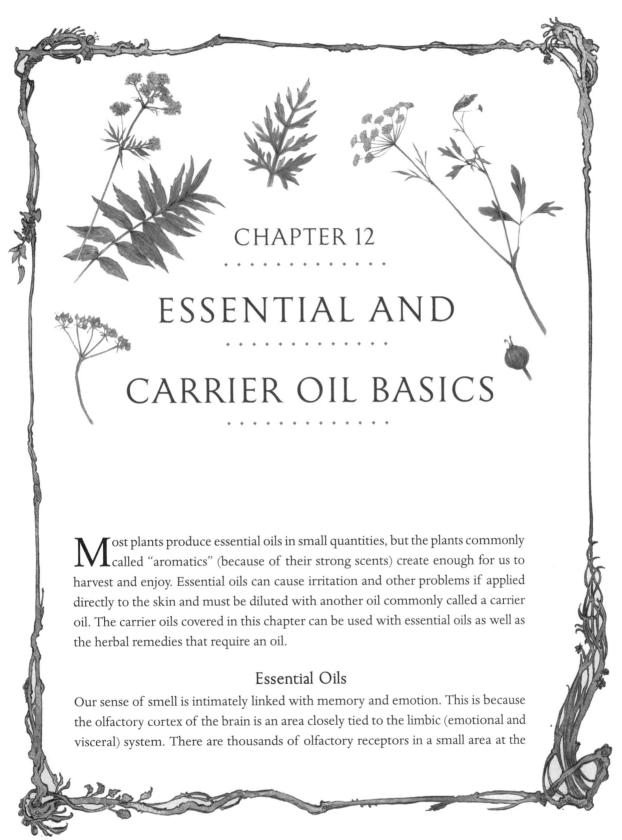

CHAPTER 12

· · · · · · · · · ·

ESSENTIAL AND

· · · · · · · · · ·

CARRIER OIL BASICS

· · · · · · · · · ·

Most plants produce essential oils in small quantities, but the plants commonly called "aromatics" (because of their strong scents) create enough for us to harvest and enjoy. Essential oils can cause irritation and other problems if applied directly to the skin and must be diluted with another oil commonly called a carrier oil. The carrier oils covered in this chapter can be used with essential oils as well as the herbal remedies that require an oil.

Essential Oils

Our sense of smell is intimately linked with memory and emotion. This is because the olfactory cortex of the brain is an area closely tied to the limbic (emotional and visceral) system. There are thousands of olfactory receptors in a small area at the top of each nasal cavity, and as we breathe in, air passes over these receptors and information is carried along a nerve into the brain. Essential oils provide immediate access to this rich storehouse of memory and emotion, which is why aromatherapy can be a powerful treatment. However, the term "aromatherapy" is a limited description of essential oil uses. They can be used topically to fight infection, heal skin problems, soothe sore muscles, and ease joint pain. In steam inhalations they can relieve congestion.

Plants produce essential oils for various functions such as aiding growth, attracting insects for pollination, and protecting against fungi or bacteria. Essential oils are obtained from various plant parts, and some plants may produce separate oils from different parts. For example, lavender essential oil is produced from the combination of leaves and flowers, whereas, angelica yields two separate oils from its seeds and roots. Essential oils are obtained from:

- leaves, stems, twigs
- flowers, flower buds
- fruit or the peel
- wood, bark
- resin, oleoresin, gum
- roots, rhizomes, bulbs
- seeds, kernels, nuts

Most of us have an idea of what an essential oil is, but the term is often mistakenly applied to a broad range of aromatic products from almost any natural source. Two key aspects to essential oils are that they dissolve in alcohol or oil but not in water, and that they evaporate when exposed to the air, which is why they are also called volatile oils. Most essential oils are liquid, but some, such as rose oil, may become a semisolid depending on the temperature. Some oils are solids. However, the defining factor is the method used to extract the oil from plant material. Essential oils are obtained through the processes of distillation and expression. Anything else is an aromatic extract, which is most often obtained by solvent extraction. The products created by solvent extraction contain both volatile and nonvolatile components.

The oldest and easiest method of oil extraction is called expression, or cold pressing. *Cold pressed* may be a familiar term for those who enjoy cooking with olive oil. For essential oils, this extraction process works only with citrus fruits because they hold high quantities of oil near the surface of their rinds. Depending on the plant, the whole fruit or just the peel is crushed and then the volatile oil is separated out using a centrifuge. This simple mechanical method does not require heat or chemicals.

The most prevalent process for extracting essential oils is through distillation, which can be accomplished using steam or water. In the distillation process, the water-soluble and water-insoluble parts of plants are separated, allowing the essential oil to be collected. Sometimes products are distilled a second time to further purify the oil and rid it of any nonvolatile material that may have been left behind the first time.

When steam is used in the distillation process, it is pumped into a vessel from underneath the plant material. Heat and pressure within the vessel, produced by the steam, causes the plant material to break down and release its volatile oil. The oil becomes vaporized and is transported with the steam through the still into a condenser, where it is cooled. This returns the oil and water to their liquid states. Depending on the density of the oil, it will either float to the top or sink to the bottom of the water. Either way, it is easily separated out. Different plants, as well as various parts of plants, require different amounts of time and temperatures for distillation.

In the water distillation process, plant material is completely immersed in hot water. This process uses less pressure and slightly lower temperatures than steam distillation. Nevertheless, for some plants, such as clary and lavender, steam distillation works better.

After the essential oil is separated from the water in these distillation processes, the water itself is an aromatic by-product called a hydrosol. Traditionally these have been called floral waters (i.e., rosewater) and contain the water-soluble molecules of aromatic plants. Hydrosols are also called hydroflorates and hydrolats. Hydrosols should never be used in place of flower essence remedies as they are not prepared under the same conditions required for consumable products.

The term "flower essence" may cause some confusion because this product is not fragrant and it is not an essential oil. A flower essence is an infusion of flowers in water, which is then mixed in a 50 percent brandy solution. Whereas the brandy acts as a preservative for flower essences, hydrosols being mostly water, can go bad. Just because flower essences contain alcohol, they should not be confused with tinctures, which are made with much higher concentrations of herbs. We will learn more about tinctures in chapter 13.

Carrier Oils for Essential Oils and Herbal Remedies

Carrier oils are also called "base" or "fixed" oils because they do not evaporate when exposed to air as essential oils do. Essential oils are very lipophilic, which means they are readily absorbed by fatty oils and waxes. Because most carrier oils are produced from the fatty portions of plants—such as seeds, kernels, or nuts—they absorb essential oils, which become diluted as they are dispersed throughout the carrier oil.

Carrier oils come from fatty plant matter, so they can go rancid if not stored properly. Like essential oils, they should be kept in dark, airtight bottles away from sun and artificial light. The shelf life of carrier oils depends on the type of oil. Storing them in the refrigerator can help keep them fresh and extend their shelf life slightly. However, like anything else we keep in the fridge, it can eventually go bad. If an oil does not look or smell right, throw it away.

Most carrier oils have their own smell, which can be sweet, nutty, herbaceous, or spicy. These are not as strong as the aromatic oils and generally do not interfere with the fragrance of essential oils. At this point, you may be thinking that the standard vegetable oil from the supermarket doesn't have any smell. This is true because chemical solvents are used to bleach and deodorize them as well as kill bacteria. While this extends the shelf life of the oil, it also means that we are putting chemicals into and onto our bodies when we use them.

When choosing an oil for making remedies, or cooking oil for that matter, select one that is unrefined and, if possible, organic. Refined oils are produced as cheaply as possible with the aid of solvents, and more and more often they are being produced from genetically modified plants. Refined oils are produced to have no odor and very little to no color. As a result, these have little nutritional or healing value. In addition, some of the plant material harvested to make these oils is often stored for a year or more before being processed. When it is finally hauled out, the raw material is washed with chemicals to remove any mold that may have grown on it while in storage.

A cycle of processes is used because after one process adds something to get rid of the oil's natural odor or color, it is followed by another process to remove whatever was put in to do the job. After wringing most of the nutrients out of the oil, it is subjected to one last process called winterizing, which keeps it from turning cloudy at lower temperatures. Unrefined oils may appear cloudy when stored in the fridge, but this does not change their chemical compositions or harm them. I prefer the clouds and shorter shelf life for my oils.

There are a number of terms applied to oils. *Partially refined* means that the oil was subjected to some of the chemical processes, which most often includes bleaching, deodorizing, and winterization. The word *pure* just means that it was not mixed with any other type of oil. The word *natural* on the label means that it was not diluted with a synthetic oil.

An unrefined oil may be labeled "cold pressed" or "expeller pressed," which means that it was not subjected to high temperatures. Plant material is usually put through a press more than once in order to squeeze out as much oil as possible. Oil that is extracted from the first pressing is called "virgin."

Commonly Used Unrefined Carrier Oils			
Oil	*Shelf Life*	*Description*	*Attributes*
Almond	12 months	Light texture; medium viscosity	Softens, soothes, and nourishes the skin; absorbs well
Apricot kernel	6–12 months	Light texture; medium viscosity	Heals dry, sensitive, inflamed, or irritated skin; easily absorbed
Avocado	12 months	Heavy texture; thick viscosity	Heals and nourishes the skin; usually mixed with a lighter oil for use
Borage seed	6 months; refrigerate	Light texture; medium viscosity	Heals and rejuvenates the skin; usually mixed with another oil for use
Coconut	1–2 years	Light texture; medium viscosity	Moisturizes and protects the skin; easily absorbed; solidifies at cool temperatures
Hemp seed	6–12 months; refrigerate	Light texture; medium viscosity	Nourishes the skin; easily absorbed
Jojoba	Up to 5 years	Heavy texture; medium viscosity when warmed; actually a wax	Excellent moisturizer, good for inflamed or irritated skin, resembles the skin's natural oil; solid at room temperature
Olive	1–2 years	Heavy texture; thick viscosity	Good for dehydrated or irritated skin; usually mixed with a lighter oil for use
Sunflower	12 months	Light texture; light viscosity	Especially good for delicate skin
Wheat germ	12 months	Heavy texture; thick viscosity	Soothes and regenerates the skin; usually mixed with a lighter oil for use

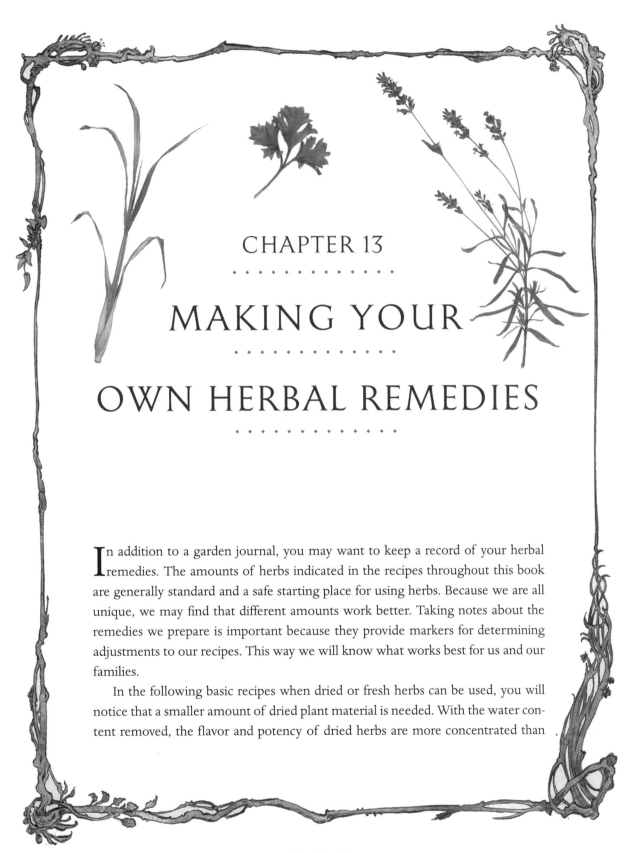

CHAPTER 13

· · · · · · · · · · · ·

MAKING YOUR

· · · · · · · · · · · · ·

OWN HERBAL REMEDIES

· · · · · · · · · · · · · ·

In addition to a garden journal, you may want to keep a record of your herbal remedies. The amounts of herbs indicated in the recipes throughout this book are generally standard and a safe starting place for using herbs. Because we are all unique, we may find that different amounts work better. Taking notes about the remedies we prepare is important because they provide markers for determining adjustments to our recipes. This way we will know what works best for us and our families.

In the following basic recipes when dried or fresh herbs can be used, you will notice that a smaller amount of dried plant material is needed. With the water content removed, the flavor and potency of dried herbs are more concentrated than fresh. When making oils, salves, ointments, butters, and honey, using dried herbs is actually better because the water content of fresh herbs can spoil the preparation. This is because water encourages the growth of bacteria and mold. If you want to use fresh herbs for these preparations, allow them to sit at room temperature for several hours until they wilt. This reduces their water content. When using frozen herbs, thaw and drain them first to reduce their water content.

Whatever preparation you make, label it with the date, the herbs that you used, and anything else that was added to it. Use glass, enamel, or stainless steel pots and pans and plastic or stainless steel sieves. Don't use aluminum utensils as this metal can be absorbed by the herbs, making them potentially toxic. Be sure that all utensils and containers for making and storing herbal remedies are clean.

The Foundation Mixtures

While these preparations serve as the base for many of the other forms of remedies discussed in the next chapter, they are also used as remedies themselves. When making preparations with seeds, toast them lightly before crushing them. To toast seeds, place them in a dry frying pan over low heat and warm them just long enough to bring out their aroma. This will enhance the flavor of your remedies and cooking.

Teas / Tisanes

Technically, "teas" are made only from the *Camellia sinensis* plant. These are the familiar black or green teas. What is commonly called an "herbal tea" is technically a mild infusion known as a tisane (pronounced tih-zahn). The word tisane comes from the Latin *ptisana*, which was a barley tea given to people during illness.[7] At any rate, because so many of us are used to calling a tisane "tea," I have kept to this convention throughout the book.

Tea can be made from various parts of plants: leaves, flowers, roots, bark, fruits, and seeds. The specific plant determines which part or parts are used. Tea made from the tougher parts, such as roots and seeds, should be steeped longer. Tea can also be made with a decoction.

Tea is usually made by the cup and consumed immediately, whereas infusions are generally made in larger amounts with some kept for later use. Also, infusions are stronger and brewed longer than tea.

When making a cup of tea, I usually add a little extra water to the kettle to allow for some boil-off. I also like to warm the cup with hot tap water for a few minutes before using it. This way the cup will not draw off some of the heat and leave the herbs to brew in tepid water. Special brewing cups with lids are available, but I find that placing a saucer over the cup works just as well.

---

7. Cynthia Black, *Natural and Herbal Family Remedies: Storey's Country Wisdom Bulletin A-168* (North Adams, MA: Storey Publishing, 1997), 13.

Basic Recipe for Tea

1–2 teaspoons dried herb, crumbled

or 2–4 teaspoons fresh herb, chopped

or 1 teaspoon decoction

per cup of boiling water

Bring the water to a boil, remove it from the heat, and let it come down slightly from the boiling point. Pour it into a cup containing the herb(s), cover, and let it steep for 10 to 20 minutes. Strain out the herbs before drinking.

....

Another tea to make is sun tea. Also called a solar infusion, sun tea is fun to make in the summer, especially if you are spending the day at the beach or the pool. Tea made this way will not be as strong as brewing it the conventional way, but it makes a healthy summer drink. Place the herbs in a jar with cold water and then put the lid on tight. Set the jar in direct sunlight for several hours. Put a couple of ice cubes in a glass, pour in some tea, and it's ready to drink.

While tea is most often consumed warm or hot, depending on the situation and herb, it can also be drunk at room temperature or chilled. The general course of treatment with tea is to drink two to four cups a day. When used as a sleep aid, drink it at least thirty minutes before going to bed. For a headache, drink the tea several times a day between meals.

Infusions

An infusion is steeped longer than a tea, and, of course, the longer it steeps, the stronger it will be. However, with some herbs, such as chamomile, a long steep brings out other qualities such as bitterness. Also, the length of time you steep it may vary according to what works best for you.

Infusions are made with the aerial parts (leaves and flowers) of a plant and sometimes with seeds or berries. The medicinal value of an infusion is that the volatile oils are captured. However, these oils can be lost if the infusion is not covered while steeping. A large jar or teapot works well for steeping infusions. When using a teapot, cover it with a dish towel to keep it warm and to block the release of steam through the spout. While it's best to make an infusion on the day you will use it, it can be stored in the fridge for a day or two.

Basic Recipe for an Infusion

4–6 tablespoons dried herb, crumbled

or 6–8 tablespoons fresh herb, chopped

per quart of boiling water

Add herb(s) to the boiling water. Steep for 30 to 45 minutes or longer according to your needs, and then strain.

....

A maceration or cold infusion is made with cold water instead of hot. Use the same amounts of herbs and water as noted above. Let the plant material soak for twelve to twenty-four hours in a cool place. Strain it and use as you would an infusion or decoction. While the decoction method is most often used for roots, a maceration works best for valerian root.

If you are not using it right away, leave the plant material in the jar while you store it for a stronger infusion. Infusions can be used instead of bath oils or salts for a therapeutic soak in the tub. When made for the bath or other external uses, infusions can be made stronger than those taken internally.

Oil Infusions

As the name implies, instead of infusing herbs in water these are steeped in oil. Infused oils are commonly used for cooking. Rosemary and garlic oils are particularly popular. Medicinal infused oils are used for massage and bath oils and for making balms, creams, salves, and ointments.

Infused oils can also be made by cold or hot methods. Making a cold infused oil is an easier but slower process. On the other hand, hot infused oils can be kept longer; sometimes for up to a year. Olive oil is often a good choice for a base oil as it rarely goes rancid. The hot infused method works best with the tougher parts of a plant such as roots, fruit, and seeds. The cold method works best with leaves and flowers, which tend to be more heat sensitive.

Basic Recipe for a Cold Oil Infusion

As with most preparations, this can be made with fresh or dried herbs. Essential oils can be used instead of plant material for an oil that will be used externally.

¼ cup dried herb, crumbled
or ¾ cup fresh herb, chopped
per pint of oil

Place the herbs in a clear glass jar and slowly pour in the oil. Gently poke around with a butter knife to release any air pockets. Leave the jar open for several hours to allow additional air to escape. If most of the oil gets absorbed, add a little more to cover the herbs. After you put the lid on the jar, gently swirl the contents. Place the jar where it will stay at room temperature for 4 to 6 weeks. Herbs left longer than this may turn moldy. Strain the oil into a dark glass bottle for storage. For a stronger oil, put new plant material into a clear glass bottle, strain the infused oil into it, and repeat the process.

When using fresh herbs, check for any condensation in the bottle after it is stored. As previously mentioned, the moisture content of fresh herbs gets released into the oil and can foster bacteria growth.

....

Basic Recipe for a Hot Oil Infusion

Use a double boiler when making hot infused oil to keep it from overheating, which affects the quality of the herbs. As with the cold-infused oil, new plant material can be used to repeat the process for a stronger oil.

¼ cup dried herb, crumbled
or ¾ cup fresh herb, chopped
per pint of oil

Place the herbs in a double boiler and add the oil. Keeping the heat as low as possible, bring the oil to a slow simmer (just a few bubbles) for 30 to 60 minutes. Remove the pot from the heat and let the oil cool. Place a stainless steel strainer lined with cheesecloth over a bowl to strain the oil. When it is done dripping, fold the cheesecloth over the plant material and press as much oil as possible from the herbs. Store the oil in dark glass bottles.

....

Infusing with Essential Oils

Because essential oils disperse easily in other oils, this type of mixture is ready to go and does not require an extended infusion time. When using an essential oil for the first time, do a test patch.

To do a patch test, put a couple of drops of essential oil on your wrist and then cover it loosely with an adhesive bandage. After a couple of hours remove the bandage and check for any redness or signs of irritation. If these occur, rinse the area with cold milk. You may try the test again at another time or on the other wrist with the essential oil diluted in a carrier oil. If you have sensitive skin, it is advisable to do a patch test only with diluted oils.

The Two Percent Solution table provides a general guideline for a 2 percent ratio of essential and carrier oils. While a 2 percent ratio is considered safe for topical applications, use a 1 percent dilution for the elderly or children, or when the oil is for use on the face. People with sensitive skin should always use a few less drops of essential oil in their mixtures.

The Two Percent Solution	
Carrier Oil	*Essential Oil*
1 teaspoon	2–3 drops
1 tablespoon	6–7 drops
1 fluid ounce	12–13 drops

Decoctions

Decoctions are generally stronger than infusions and are made with the tougher, more fibrous parts of plants such as roots, bark, twigs, berries, seeds, and nuts. An exception to this is valerian root, which is actually better when prepared as a maceration instead of a decoction.

When making a decoction, fresh or dried plant material can be used. It must be chopped or broken into small pieces. Berries, seeds, and nuts should be crushed. Leaves and flowers are sometimes used in decoctions, however, these should be added just before it is finished simmering. Store a decoction in the fridge where it will keep for two or three days. For a more concentrated herbal remedy, use more plant material. A decoction can be administered hot or cold.

BASIC RECIPE FOR A DECOCTION
4–6 tablespoons dried herb, crumbled
or 6–8 tablespoons fresh herb, chopped
per quart of water

Place the plant material in a saucepan, add the water, and bring to a boil. Reduce the heat and simmer for 30 to 45 minutes or until the liquid is reduced to about one third. Let it cool, strain it into a jar, and then store it in the fridge.

Tinctures

Stronger than infusions and decoctions, tinctures are usually made with alcohol instead of water or oil. Vodka, gin, brandy, and rum work well for tinctures. Rum is particularly good to mask the taste of bitter herbs. Industrial, methyl, or isopropyl alcohols should never be used to make a tincture. Because tinctures are concentrated, they are administered in very small doses. In addition, they can be used as the base for a syrup. Tinctures should not be used during pregnancy or by anyone with gastric inflammation.

Basic Recipe for a Tincture
¾ cup dried herb, crumbled
or 1 ½ cups fresh herb, chopped
per pint of 80 to 100 proof alcohol

Place the herbs in a jar, pour in the alcohol to cover the plant material, close, and shake for 1 to 2 minutes. Set aside for 2 to 4 weeks, shaking the jar every other day. Strain out the herbs and store in dark glass bottles in a cool, dark place.

....

A tincture will keep up to two years. Another way to make a tincture is to place enough dried herbs to fill one third to one half of a pint jar. When using fresh herbs, fill the jar to three quarters or slightly more. Pour in enough alcohol to cover the herbs and follow the directions as above.

A standard tincture dose is one teaspoon, two or three times a day diluted in an ounce of water, tea, or fruit juice. Alternatively, add one teaspoon of tincture to a cup of boiling water and then wait about five minutes for the alcohol to evaporate. Tinctures can also be used straight by putting ten to fifteen drops under the tongue.

While it is not as potent, apple cider or apple cider vinegar can be substituted as a tincture base for anyone who prefers not to use alcohol. Cider or vinegar tinctures should steep for about six weeks before straining. However, they will not keep as long as those made with alcohol. Doses for these types of tinctures can be administered by sprinkling on a salad.

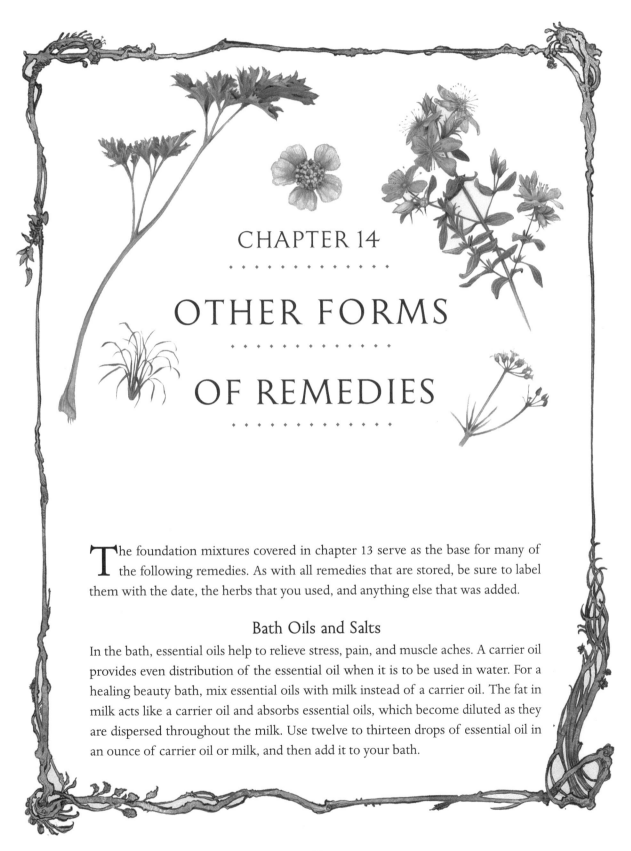

CHAPTER 14

· · · · ·

OTHER FORMS

· · · · ·

OF REMEDIES

· · · · ·

The foundation mixtures covered in chapter 13 serve as the base for many of the following remedies. As with all remedies that are stored, be sure to label them with the date, the herbs that you used, and anything else that was added.

Bath Oils and Salts

In the bath, essential oils help to relieve stress, pain, and muscle aches. A carrier oil provides even distribution of the essential oil when it is to be used in water. For a healing beauty bath, mix essential oils with milk instead of a carrier oil. The fat in milk acts like a carrier oil and absorbs essential oils, which become diluted as they are dispersed throughout the milk. Use twelve to thirteen drops of essential oil in an ounce of carrier oil or milk, and then add it to your bath.

In addition to carrier oils and milk, essential oils can be mixed with salts. Epsom salts are healing on their own and make a good medium for essential oils. Coarse sea salt can also be used. Salts contain minerals that aid in the release of toxins from the muscles and joints, which is beneficial when dealing with infectious illnesses, rheumatism, and arthritis. Of course, salts also promote relaxation.

Basic Recipe for Bath Salts

2 cups Epsom or sea salts

2 tablespoons baking soda (optional)

10–15 drops essential oil

Place the dry ingredients in a glass bowl. Add the essential oil and mix thoroughly. Store the bath salts in a jar with a tight lid. The optional baking soda helps to soothe the skin. To use the salts, add a handful or two under the running tap to dissolve them.

Compresses

Compresses can be used hot or cold. Warm compresses relax muscles and soothe aches and pains. They also relieve tension and increase circulation. Cold compresses are used to treat bumps, bruises, and sprains by reducing swelling and inflammation. They also reduce fevers and ease headaches.

A tea or infusion of herbs can be used to soak a face cloth that is then squeezed out and laid over the area that needs treatment. Alternatively, 5 or 6 drops of essential oil in a tablespoon of carrier oil can be added to 1 quart of hot or cold water. Give the water a swish before dipping in the cloth. Whichever method is used, the cloth should be dipped in the infusion or water with essential oil to freshen it every ten to fifteen minutes.

Fomentation

Alternating warm and cold compresses is a remedy called fomentation. It is used to manipulate the flow of blood in an area of the body. Start with a hot compress for about five minutes to relax and open the capillaries. Follow with a cold compress, which causes the capillaries to constrict and push blood out of the area. Leave the cold compress on for two or three minutes. Replace the cold compress with a fresh warm compress, which will open the capillaries again, bringing fresh blood into the affected area. Continue alternating the compresses for fifteen to twenty minutes. This is especially helpful for treating low back pain, muscle strains, and kidney stones.

Creams

A cream is a combination of oils and an herbal infusion that nourishes and heals the skin as it is absorbed. Shea butter and a little bit of beeswax serve as the base to thicken the mixture and give it a creamy consistency. The amount of shea butter, beeswax, and oil may vary according to your preference.

The easiest way to make a cream is to use a mason jar in a saucepan of water that is at least half as deep as the jar is tall. The instructions on how to make a cream provides two sets of ingredients: one is for making the cream with an herbal infusion; the second is for making it with essential oil.

BASIC RECIPES FOR CREAM

Ingredients using herbal infusion	Ingredients using essential oil
½ cup shea butter	½ cup shea butter
2–3 beeswax pastilles (pellets)	2–3 beeswax pastilles (pellets)
½ cup almond, coconut, or other oil	½ cup almond, coconut, or other oil
1 cup herbal infusion	1 cup distilled or filtered water
	2 teaspoons essential oil

Place the shea butter and beeswax pastilles in the jar and warm over low heat. When the butter and beeswax begin to melt, add the oil and stir gently with a fork. When everything has melted, remove from the heat and stir. Let the mixture cool slightly, pour it into a blender, and add either the herbal infusion or the water and essential oil. Whip it to get a light, creamy consistency. You may need to experiment with the amount of oil to get a consistency you like. Transfer the cream to a jar, allow it to cool, and then store.

Diffusers and Vaporizers

Diffusers and vaporizers provide the means to disperse essential oils into the air. Vaporizers are usually ceramic with a small bowl on top and a space for a tea light candle underneath. It works by placing a few drops of essential oil in the bowl, which is then warmed by the candle flame. As it warms, the essential oil will evaporate. Diffusers are electronic, which makes them safer than candles for heating oil, especially if you want to use it at night or in a child's room. Most diffusers have settings to adjust the rate of evaporation.

Obviously, this scents the air and is generally what comes to mind when we think of aromatherapy. While it is a great way to use lavender or other essential oils to relieve stress and enhance well-being, there is much more to it. Essential oils with antiseptic qualities also kill airborne bacteria. Because essential oils in the air are absorbed into the body, oils that fight infection or relieve congestion can be used this way. It is a good way to fight colds and flu, and to treat asthma or bronchitis. In addition, some oils can help repel insects, making this an ideal way to use them in the summer.

Reed Diffusers

A gentle, safe, and off-the-grid method is to use a reed diffuser. It takes a little longer to disperse the essential oil into the air, but it is a nice alternative to commercial air fresheners. There are just a few things you will need to make a reed diffuser:

- A glass or porcelain container
- Reeds
- Carrier oil
- Essential oil(s)

A short glass or porcelain jar or a vase with a narrow neck works best. Plastic should be avoided as chemicals from the plastic container can leach into the oils. A wide-mouthed jar with a cork can be adjusted by drilling a hole in the cork so it is large enough to accommodate the reeds. There are several types of reeds on the market, however, rattan reeds work best as they are porous and wick the oils more evenly. The reeds should be at least twice the height of the jar.

Choose a light carrier oil for the base as thicker ones are not drawn up the reeds as easily. Sweet almond oil is often recommended, but I have found that sunflower, being a very thin oil, works best. If you are using more than one essential oil, blend those together first and then give them about a week for the combined scent to mature.

Pour ¼ cup of carrier oil into your diffuser jar, add 2 teaspoons of the essential oil or oil blend, and swirl to mix. Place the reeds in the jar and turn them a couple of times the first day to diffuse the scent. After that, turn them once a day or every other day. Over time, you will need to add more oil to the jar. When the reeds become saturated, replace them.

There are several things to avoid when making a reed diffuser. First, the fragrance oils on the market for reed diffusers are synthetic and not essential oils. Some of them may smell nice, but they are made from chemicals, not plants. The commercial base oils for reed diffusers are also usually chemical-based. Mineral oil and dipropylene glycol are sometimes recommended as a base but avoid these for the same reason.

Foot Soaks

Infusions and essential oils, either diluted in a carrier oil or bath salts, can be used for footbaths. A warm or hot footbath increases circulation, aids in healing a cold or flu, and helps deal with insomnia. Odd as it may seem, a foot soak helps relieve headaches. Even soaking your feet in plain warm water helps to draw blood down to the feet, which relieves pressure in the head. A cool foot bath is a good perk-up on hot summer days when feet can be sweaty and sore.

Liniments

Like a tincture, a liniment is made with alcohol, however, a liniment is for external application only and should never be taken internally. A liniment is used to relieve the pain of stiff joints, sore muscles, strains, and sprains. It also aids in healing bruises and disinfecting wounds. A warming liniment can be made with cayenne to relieve pain and stiffness; a cooling liniment can be made with peppermint to reduce swelling and inflammation. To use a liniment, rub it onto the affected area or saturate a washcloth to use as a compress.

Rubbing alcohol, or isopropyl alcohol, is often recommended as the base for a liniment and is very effective. However, it can dry the skin, and for some people it can be an irritant. Witch hazel makes a good liniment base as it contains a low amount of alcohol. As an alternative, use witch hazel water and isopropyl alcohol so you can mix them and control the amount of alcohol in the liniment. White vinegar can also be used as a liniment base. Be sure to label your liniment for external use only.

BASIC RECIPE FOR A LINIMENT

4 tablespoons herb

1 pint alcohol, witch hazel, or other base

Place the herbs in a jar and pour in the alcohol. Set aside for 4 to 6 weeks, giving the jar a good shake every day. Strain, then store in a dark bottle.

....

Medicinal Honey

Honey is a good way to administer herbal remedies, especially to children. Quite simply, it is an infusion made with honey instead of water or oil. There are two ways to make a medicinal honey. The herbs can be crushed or chopped and put directly into the honey or they can be tied into a piece of cheesecloth or muslin for easy removal. Herbs placed directly into the honey can be strained out before storage or left in. Fresh herbs should be removed before storage because of their water content.

BASIC RECIPE FOR A MEDICINAL HONEY

½ cup dried herb, crumbled

or ¾ cup fresh herb, chopped

per cup of honey

Pour the honey into a slightly larger mason jar and set it in a saucepan of water that is at least half as deep as the jar is tall. Warm it over low heat until the honey becomes a little less viscous, and then add the herbs or herb sack. Use a butter knife to stir loose herbs throughout the honey or to push the herb sack down so it is covered. Continue warming for 15 to 20 minutes. Remove from the heat, set aside, and when it is cool put the lid on the jar. Store out of the light at room temperature for a week.

If you are going to remove the herbs, heat the honey again and then strain it into a new jar or remove the herb sack. Squeeze the herb sack to get as much honey as you can out of it. The honey can be stored in a cupboard for up to 18 months. A spoonful of honey can be used in tea or taken straight.

....

Things to Know When Buying Honey

When purchasing honey, there are a number of things to keep in mind, especially for medicinal uses. Words like "pure" and "natural" on honey labels sound good; however, unlike "organic" there are no government standards for these classifications. In addition, the czars of marketing would have us believe that good honey is golden and clear but this is not usually the case. Honey can range in color from very light to dark mahogany and in consistency from watery to thick to crystallized. Like taste and aroma, the color depends on the plants and flowers the bees have dined upon.

Good honey is cloudy, not clear. This is because of its pollen content, which gives honey its valuable enzymes, vitamins, minerals, and antioxidants. A traditional filtering process catches bee parts, wax, and debris from the hives but leaves the pollen in the honey.

The problem is that retailers want a product that has a long shelf life and many packers want to use the cheapest honey to increase their profit margins. A commonly-used process called "ultra filtering" not only heats and waters down the honey but also removes the pollen. In addition to taking away this healthy component, removing the pollen removes the only way to identify the source of the honey. There is no way to tell if the honey came from a country with low standards and regulations regarding pesticides or from a country where pollution and contamination may be a problem. To make matters worse, some honey has additives such as corn syrup.

The best sources for good honey are local beekeepers or local farmers markets. If that doesn't work for you, try health food stores or supermarkets where you can get organic honey. Read the labels to be sure you are buying honey and not a honey-flavored product.

Also, be critical. For example, a monofloral honey can be quite nice and it is often expensive. Monofloral is a type of honey where the predominant flavor and pollen comes from one type of flower. Unfortunately, this can be faked. One time I was excited to find a lavender honey less expensive than expected only to read the label and discover that instead of a monofloral honey, lavender essential oil had been added. Needless to say, I did not buy this deceptive product.

When it comes to storing honey, it is best to keep it at room temperature and not in the fridge or cool cabinet. Also, like many foods, it is better to store honey in a glass jar rather than plastic. Unfortunately, it is best to part company with the little plastic squeeze bear.

Ointments, Salves, and Balms

Ointments, salves, and balms are basically the same but differ by the amount of solidifier, such as beeswax, used to thicken them. An ointment is the least firm with the consistency of pudding. The advantage of an ointment is that it is easy to apply. A salve has a firmer consistency, and a balm is very firm. Unlike a cream, these preparations are not absorbed as much and form a protective layer on the skin.

The solidifier for these preparations can be beeswax or jojoba. The instructions on how to make these preparations provides two sets of ingredients. One is for making them with an infused oil; the second is for making them with essential oil. These preparations will keep for several months to a year.

BASIC RECIPES FOR OINTMENTS, SALVES, AND BALMS

Ingredients using an infused oil	*Ingredients using essential oil*
¼–½ cup beeswax or jojoba	¼–½ cup beeswax or jojoba
1 cup infused oil	1 cup carrier oil
	2 teaspoons essential oil

Place the jojoba or beeswax in a mason jar in a saucepan of water that is at least half as deep as the jar is tall. Warm it over low heat, and when it begins to melt, add the infused oil. Stir gently with a fork for about 15 minutes. If you are making it with essential oil, add the carrier oil on its own as you would the infused oil. Add the essential oil when you remove the jar from the heat and stir.

To test the thickness, spoon a little of the mixture onto a plate and put it in the refrigerator for a minute or two to cool. Check the thickness. If you want it firmer, add more of the solidifying ingredient. If it's too thick, add a tiny bit of oil. When you are happy with the consistency of your preparation, let it cool, and then store in a cool, dark place.

....

Poultices

A poultice is an herb paste that is applied to an affected area. It can be used to ease muscle or nerve pain, insect bites, rashes, burns, and swollen glands. A poultice draws impurities out of infected wounds or boils. It must be made fresh each time it is needed.

BASIC RECIPE FOR FRESH HERB POULTICE

½ cup fresh herb, chopped

1 cup boiling water

Chop and mash the herbs before adding them to the water. Stir and let simmer for 1 to 2 minutes. Let it cool and then strain the liquid away to make a paste.

....

Basic Recipe for Dried Herb Poultice

1–2 tablespoons dried herb, crumbled

enough water to moisten

Crumble or grind 1 or 2 tablespoons of dried herbs. Boil water and add just enough to moisten the herbs to make a paste.

....

When the poultice is cool enough to handle, cover the skin with gauze and spoon a sufficient amount of the poultice on so it covers the affected area with a thick ¼- to ½-inch layer. Cover with another piece of gauze to keep the poultice in place, and then put a towel over it to keep the warmth in. Remove the poultice when it becomes cool. Apply a poultice 1 to 3 times a day, making it fresh each time.

Powders and Capsules

A blender, food processor, or flour mill can be used to create an herb powder from dried herbs. Store the powder in a tightly closed glass jar out of sunlight. Powders can be used to make herbal butters and breads and as a seasoning for food. Powders can be mixed into other preparations and some can be used for first aid.

In powdered form, herbs can be taken in capsules, which is easier if you do not like the taste of a particular herb. Valerian is one such plant that many people prefer to ingest in capsules. Gelatin and vegetarian capsule cases are readily available in many health food stores and online. Capsule size "00" is commonly used for powdered herbs. Two capsules are considered a standard dose for adults. One capsule holds approximately 250 milligrams.

The most important thing when filling capsules is to have dry hands, otherwise the capsules will stick to your fingers. There are two halves to a capsule: one is longer and slightly narrower (the bottom); the other is shorter and slightly wider (the cap) to fit over the bottom half. To fill, sprinkle a small mound of powder on a saucer and scoop as much powder as you can into the bottom half of the capsule.

Another way to fill them is to use a small piece of paper to make a tiny funnel so you can pour the powder into the bottom half. Either way, when you get as much herb powder into the capsule as you can, slide the halves together. Store capsules in a dark, airtight glass container in a cool place.

Sleep Pillows

If you want the advantages of herbal aromas at night but don't want to leave a diffuser running, a sleep pillow is a good option. A sleep pillow is a small pillow stuffed with herbs that is placed beside your regular pillow at night. You don't even need a sewing machine to make one as they can be stitched by hand.

Five inches square is a good size, but you can make one bigger or smaller or in any shape. Cotton fabric is easy to work with and is available in many colors and designs. Choose something that you find soothing.

Fold the fabric in half with the "right" sides (the side with the pattern, darker design, or color) facing each other. Pin the fabric to hold it together. Using a ruler and pencil, measure and draw the shape of the pillow, making it about half an inch larger than the finished size on all sides. That will be your cut line. Draw another line half an inch inside the cut line to serve as your sewing line. Using scissors, follow the first line you drew to cut the fabric. Stitch around all sides (assuming the pillow is a square or rectangle), leaving a two-inch opening on one side. Turn the fabric inside out through the opening, putting the stitching and unfinished edges of fabric inside. The brighter color or design of the fabric will be on the outside. Stuff the pillow with dried herbs, and then tuck the edges of the opening inside and stitch it closed.

A sleep pillow can be freshened from time to time with a couple of drops of essential oil. When not in use, store the pillow in a plastic bag or container so the herbs will continue to infuse the fabric with their aroma and hold the fragrance. Warming the pillow in a microwave before use helps bring out more fragrance.

Steam Inhalations

Because steam and antiseptic ingredients help clear the respiratory airways, it is a good way to treat congested sinuses as well as chest infections. Facial steams for the skin help to deep clean pores and add moisture. The combination of steam and herbs or essential oils is also a good way to cleanse the air of a sickroom and to humidify or freshen a room in the winter.

The recipe for making a steam inhalation provides two sets of ingredients. One is for making it with herbs, and the second is for making it with essential oil. Because the essential oil is not going to be used directly on the skin, diluting it in a carrier oil is not necessary.

BASIC RECIPES FOR A STEAM INHALATION

Ingredients using herbs	Ingredients using essential oil
1 quart water	1 quart water
7 tablespoons dried herbs	5–10 drops essential oil

Add the herbs to boiling water and simmer on low heat for 5 minutes. If you are using essential oil, add it to the water after removing it from the heat.

....

For a facial steam or when treating respiratory problems, place a bath towel over your head to create a tent above the steaming water. Keep your eyes closed and don't move your face too close to the water. Stay under the tent for three minutes or until the water cools. If it feels too hot, lift the towel to allow cool air into the tent.

If you are using it to cleanse and humidify the air, place the saucepan in the room where it is needed. When it cools, the mixture can be reheated for more steam.

Syrups

Syrups are soothing and good for treating sore throats as well as coughs. They are also an easy way to take medicine. A dose is usually one teaspoon. Syrups can be made with dried herbs, a tincture, infusion, or decoction. When making a syrup with dried herbs, you may need to adjust the amount of honey to get a syrup consistency that you like.

BASIC RECIPE FOR A SYRUP USING DRIED HERBS

4 tablespoons dried herbs, crumbled

½ cup honey

1 quart water

Put the herbs in a saucepan of water and bring it to a simmer. Keep it on low heat until the volume is reduced to a little less than half. Strain out the herbs, return the liquid to the saucepan, and add the honey. Warm it on low heat, stirring until the mixture is smooth. Let it cool a little and then pour it into a jar. Store in the fridge where it will keep for several weeks.

....

BASIC RECIPE FOR A SYRUP USING A TINCTURE

2–4 tablespoons tincture

1 cup honey

Warm the honey in a double boiler over low heat. Add the tincture and continue heating it on low for 10 to 15 minutes. Let it cool, and then bottle it and store in the fridge for up to 6 months.

....

BASIC RECIPE FOR A SYRUP USING AN INFUSION OR DECOCTION

⅔ cup infusion or decoction

⅓ cup honey

Combine the ingredients in a saucepan. Stir over low heat until the honey is less viscous and the mixture is smooth. Cool and store in the fridge. It will keep for several weeks.

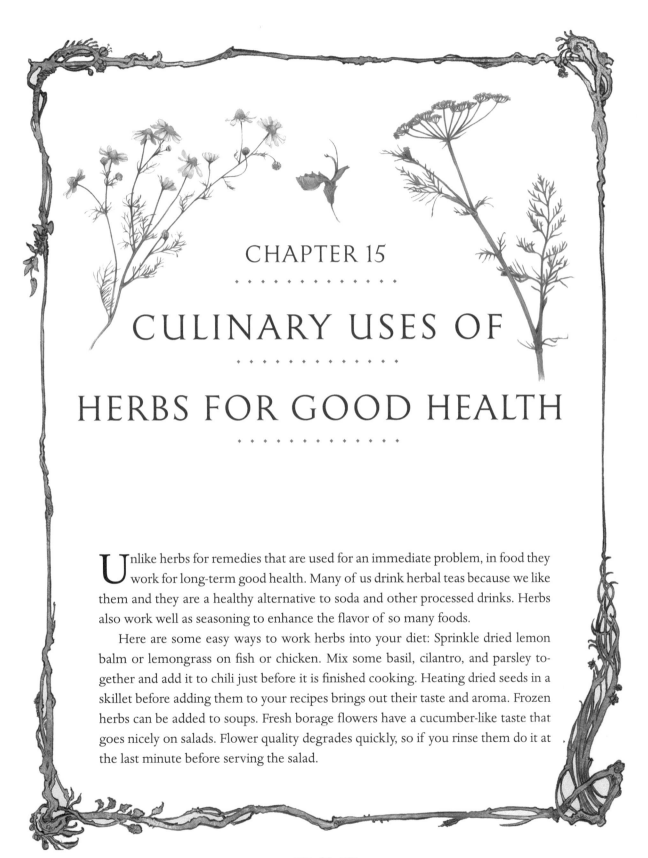

CHAPTER 15

· · · · · · · · · ·

CULINARY USES OF

· · · · · · · · · · ·

HERBS FOR GOOD HEALTH

· · · · · · · · · ·

Unlike herbs for remedies that are used for an immediate problem, in food they work for long-term good health. Many of us drink herbal teas because we like them and they are a healthy alternative to soda and other processed drinks. Herbs also work well as seasoning to enhance the flavor of so many foods.

Here are some easy ways to work herbs into your diet: Sprinkle dried lemon balm or lemongrass on fish or chicken. Mix some basil, cilantro, and parsley together and add it to chili just before it is finished cooking. Heating dried seeds in a skillet before adding them to your recipes brings out their taste and aroma. Frozen herbs can be added to soups. Fresh borage flowers have a cucumber-like taste that goes nicely on salads. Flower quality degrades quickly, so if you rinse them do it at the last minute before serving the salad.

Breads

There's nothing like the smell of fresh-baked bread. Herbs enhance the aroma as well as the taste. As with many recipes, it is important to experiment to find what suits your taste. Frozen herbs need to be thawed and drained, which is especially important for biscuits and breads where extra moisture may have a detrimental impact on the recipe.

Here are the amounts of herbs to add to your dough per loaf or dozen biscuits as a starting point.

BASIC RECIPE TO ADD TO DOUGH
1 teaspoon strong-flavored fresh herbs, chopped
or 2 teaspoons mild-flavored fresh herbs, chopped
or ½ teaspoon dried herbs, crumbled

Once the dough is made, simply work the herbs into it. Herbs can be added to ready-made dough, too. Simply work the herbs into the dough. Herbs can be sprinkled onto crescent rolls before rolling them up or for pre-formed rolls just make a depression in the top of each one with your finger and sprinkle in some herbs.

....

When making bread or biscuits for a particular meal, plan to use herbs that go with the main course. For example, biscuits with parsley, sage, rosemary, or thyme go well with a turkey dinner. Don't limit herbs to breads. A simple pound cake comes to life with lemon balm, anise, or angelica. In fact, anything you bake can be enhanced with herbs. Just follow your taste buds.

Butter, Margarine, and Ghee

An herbal butter, margarine, or ghee can make any meal special. Although most recipes call for sweet, unsalted butter, taste is in the mouth of the beholder, so use what you find most pleasing. Margarine can be used instead of butter and has the advantage of usually being soft right from the fridge. Ghee is a type of clarified butter used in Indian dishes and is becoming more popular in the United States. It is created by slowly heating butter to coax and strain out the water and milk solids. Ghee usually does not need refrigeration.

BASIC RECIPE FOR HERBAL BUTTER, MARGARINE, OR GHEE
1–1½ teaspoons dried herbs, crumbled
or 1 tablespoon fresh herbs, chopped
or ½ teaspoon seeds, crushed
½ cup butter, margarine, or ghee

If you are using butter, let it stand at room temperature until it is soft. Use a fork to cream the butter or margarine so it is malleable. Add the herbs and mix until they are dispersed throughout. Spoon into a container and refrigerate until needed. When using ghee, sprinkle the herbs into the jar and mix well with a butter knife.

....

Cooking Oils

Unlike adding herbs during the cooking process, infusing an oil gives the herbs time to blend flavors with the oil. The oil also absorbs vitamins, minerals, and other nutritional components from the herbs. An infused cooking oil is great for salads, salad dressings, sauces, marinades, and a drizzle for bread, which is why they are so popular. An infused oil made with dried herbs is more stable and will last longer. In the winter, try a combination of rosemary and thyme, which tastes great while helping to prevent colds and flu.

BASIC RECIPE FOR INFUSED COOKING OIL

¼ cup dried herbs, crumbled

or ¾ cup fresh herbs, chopped

1 cup oil

Place the herbs in a jar and pour in the oil, making sure the herbs are completely covered. Let it sit for 4 weeks, shaking occasionally to mix the herbs throughout the oil. Dried herbs can be left in or strained out. Fresh herbs need to be strained out because of their water content, which can foster bacteria growth.

....

Honey

While honey is a sweetener, it is far better than sugar or the vast range of artificial sweeteners. Honey has antiseptic and antibacterial properties, and it is an aid to seasonal allergies. (Read the section in chapter 14 called "Things to Know When Buying Honey.") As you will notice, a seasoned honey generally has less herbs than a medicinal one, however, listen to your taste buds and experiment to find what suits you.

BASIC RECIPE FOR HERBAL HONEY

¼ cup dried herbs, crumbled

or ½ cup fresh herbs, chopped

1 cup honey

Pour the honey into a slightly larger mason jar and set it in a saucepan of water that is at least half as deep as the jar is tall. Warm it over low heat until the honey becomes a little less viscous, and then add the herbs or herb sack. Use a butter knife to stir loose herbs throughout the honey or to push the herb sack down so it is covered. Continue warming for 15 to 20 minutes. Remove from the heat, set aside, and when it is cool put the lid on the jar. Store it out of the light in a cupboard at room temperature for a week.

....

For a nice combination of herbal honey to add to a bedtime cup of chamomile tea, use two tablespoons of dried lavender flowers and one teaspoon of dried lemon balm leaves per cup honey.

Vinegars

Just as oils can be infused with herbs, so too can vinegar. Also like oil, vinegar absorbs vitamins and minerals from the herbs and enhances the nutritional value of food. Herbal vinegars can perk up salads, dressings, sauces, and marinades. Occasionally, herbal vinegars can be used as remedies. White or red wine vinegars tend to work best with most herbs; an exception being cider vinegar for dill. As with most things culinary, it is a matter of taste so don't be shy about experimenting.

An important thing to note about vinegar is that it reacts with most metals. Use stainless steel, glass, ceramic, or porcelain saucepans and containers. For storage, use jars and bottles with cork stoppers or plastic lids. A regular mason jar with a metal lid can be used but place two pieces of wax paper over the jar before putting on the lid.

BASIC RECIPE FOR HERBAL VINEGAR
¾ jar fresh herbs, chopped
or ¼ jar dried herbs, crushed
enough vinegar to cover the herbs

Warm the vinegar slightly. Place the herbs in a jar and pour in the vinegar. Cover and store in a cool, dark place for 2 to 4 weeks. Shake the jar a couple of times a week. As with oil, dried herbs can be left in but fresh ones need to be strained out. Store away from heat and light.

....

The use of herbs in cooking is endless and experimenting with different combinations is rewarding and tasty. Cooking with herbs is also a great way to enjoy the bounty of your garden all year.

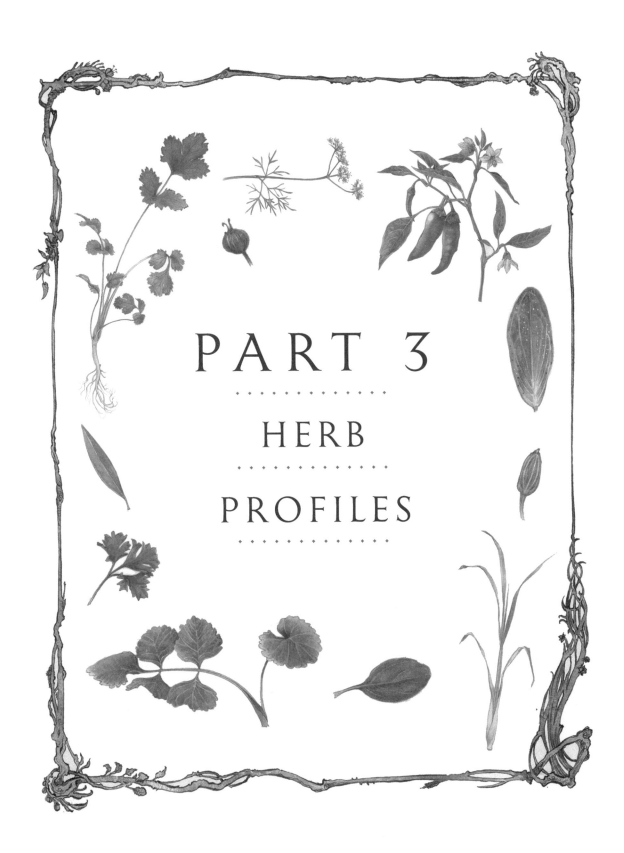

PART 3

· · · · · · · · · · · ·

HERB

· · · · · · · · · · · ·

PROFILES

· · · · · · · · · · · ·

While the basic details for making teas, infusions, creams, and other preparations is included throughout this part of the book, it's a good idea to read the full details in part 2. Likewise, some information for harvesting and preparing herbs for use is included here where specific details pertain to certain herbs. Complete instructions on harvesting and preparing herbs are also in part 2.

The recipes included here indicate either dried or fresh ingredients, however, unless otherwise noted, these are interchangeable and depend on what you have available. Check part 2 for standard amounts of herbs to use while preparing remedies. Where combinations of herbs are suggested, review the precaution information for each herb.

Plant descriptions are included in the gardening section of each herb profile. Without going into a great deal of botany, a few terms are helpful to know. Starting with leaves, some may have "lobes" and others may be "toothed." A lobed leaf has deeply indented edges, such as oak or maple tree leaves. A toothed leaf has jagged edges. Many of the leaves described here are "simple," meaning that a leaf stem has one leaf. Others are called "pinnate" leaves, which means that a leaf stem has three or more leaflets.

Where flowers are concerned, a common flower cluster structure is called an "umbel"—think umbrella. In fact both words are derived from the Latin *umbella*, "sunshade," which is a diminutive of *umbra*, meaning "shade." [8] An umbel has a number of flower stems, nearly equal in length, that spread from a common center stalk. The cluster can be flat-topped or spherical. Queen Anne's lace is an example of an umbel structure. Finally, the crown of a plant is the upper part of the root system that extends above ground.

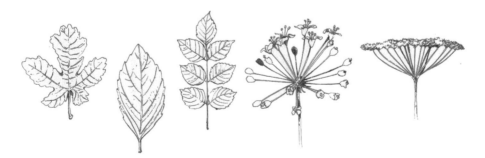

Figure 3.1: Leaves can be lobed, toothed, or pinnate.
Umbel flower structures can be spherical or flat-topped.

---

8. Ian Brookes, *Chambers Concise Dictionary* (Edinburgh, Scotland: Chambers Harrap, 2004), 1321.

Angelica

(*Angelica archangelica* L., syn. *A. officinalis*)

Also known as: Angelic Herb, Archangel, European Angelica, Garden Angelica, Wild Celery

This plant's name tells us that it is associated with angels. The connection comes from a story that mentioned this herb blooming on May 8, the feast day of St. Michael the Archangel. Its medieval Latin name was *Herba Angelica*. In 1665, a monk is said to have had a dream in which he was visited by an angel who told him that the plant could cure the plague, which was raging at that time.[9]

Angelica was a prized medicinal herb for centuries and was used in a range of remedies up through the Middle Ages and Renaissance. In the tropics, the essential oil of angelica was mixed with quinine for a more potent treatment of malaria. By the late seventeenth century, angelica's wide use as a medicinal herb declined, although it was still common in home remedies in England into the early twentieth century. In addition to medicine, this plant has been used to create green dyes.

Today angelica is highly valued as a fragrance in many commercial products as well as a flavor component in Benedictine, gin, and vermouth. It is often used as an ornamental plant because of its striking appearance.

Medicinal Uses

Amenorrhea, anorexia, anxiety, appetite stimulant, arthritis, bronchitis, cardiovascular system support, chest congestion, colds, cough, expectorant, flatulence, gastritis, headache, heartburn, indigestion, irritable bowel syndrome (IBS), menstrual cramps, menstrual cycle problems, nervous tension, psoriasis, rheumatism, skin care, stomachache or pain, stomach ulcer, stress, water retention

Precautions and Contraindications

The herb: Avoid during pregnancy; diabetics should also avoid angelica.

The essential oils: Herbal precautions apply to both essential oils. The essential oil from the root causes photosensitivity.

Parts of Plant Used

Herbal remedies: Leaves, seeds, and roots

Essential oils: Seeds and roots are used for two separate oils

Culinary purposes: Leaves, stalks, roots, and seeds

---

9. Claire Kowalchik and William H. Hylton, eds., *Rodale's Illustrated Encyclopedia of Herbs* (Emmaus, PA: Rodale Press, 1998), 10.

Growing and Harvesting

At five to eight feet tall, angelica is best described as statuesque. Its hollow stalks are round and purplish with branching stems. It has broad, pinnate leaves with coarsely toothed edges. Tiny honey-scented, white or greenish flowers grow in globe-shaped umbels that bloom mid to late summer of the second or third year. The seeds are pale, brownish-yellow when ripe and up to a quarter inch long. They are ribbed on one side. The yellowish-gray root is long, thick, and fleshy.

Type	Zone	Light	Soil	Moisture	Height	Spacing
Biennial	4	Partial shade	Loam	Moderately moist	5–8'	3'

Although angelica prefers partial shade, it is not fussy and will grow in sun or shade. It can be propagated by sowing fresh seeds or let it help you as it readily self-seeds. The plant dies back in the winter like a perennial. In fact, angelica has been called a biennial-perennial as well as a short-lived perennial because it often lives for three years. If you are planning to use different parts of this herb, you will need several plants.

Roots can be harvested in the autumn of the first year. Collect seeds in late summer of the second or third year. On the plants you are not growing for seed, cut off the flower stalks to extend the season for harvesting leaves. The leaves can be hung to air dry but do best when dried on a screen. The leaves and stalks are best when harvested in the spring of the second season. The stalks can also be frozen.

How to Use the Herb

Angelica may taste like a treat, but it is an aid to many types of digestive problems. All parts of the plant relieve indigestion and flatulence. A tea made from the leaves is the easiest preparation for dealing with these issues.

ANGEL FOR THE STOMACH ANGELICA TEA

1–2 teaspoons dried leaves, crumbled

1 cup boiling water

Combine the herb and water. Steep for 10 to 15 minutes, strain, and drink.

The tea or an infusion of leaves helps soothe stomach ulcers. For heartburn or stomachache, make the tea a little stronger by using 2 teaspoons of dried leaves or take ½ to 1 teaspoon of tincture. A decoction of the roots or seeds can also be used to treat indigestion and flatulence as well as gastritis and irritable bowel syndrome (IBS). To stimulate the appetite and aid in treating anorexia, take ¼ to ½ teaspoon of root tincture three times a day. The antispasmodic and diuretic properties of angelica make it helpful in easing menstrual cramps and relieving water retention.

WOMEN'S MONTHLY RELIEF ANGELICA TEA

1 teaspoon angelica root, chopped

½ teaspoon caraway seeds, crushed

½ teaspoon coriander seeds, crushed

1 cup boiling water

The root should be chopped into small pieces. Combine the herbs and add the water. Steep for 15 to 20 minutes and strain. Add a little honey to taste.

An infusion of angelica leaves or a decoction of the root can aid with amenorrhea or help stimulate a late menstrual cycle. Drink two or three cups of the infusion or decoction a day, or make a tincture and take a ¼ teaspoon four times a day.

Angelica root is a warming tonic for relieving cold symptoms, plus, the root has expectorant properties that help clear congestion. Drink ½ to 1 cup of root decoction when a cold first hits. For bronchitis and chest coughs, take a ¼ to ½ teaspoon of root tincture three times a day. Angelica tea made with the leaves or a decoction of the root will also help soothe a cough.

A quick way to freshen a room, especially after sickness, is with angelica incense. Simply burn a few seeds or small pieces of dried root in a metal or heat-resistant container.

All parts of angelica have a mild, spicy licorice flavor. The fresh leaves can be used in green salads, savory soups, or stews. Dried and ground, they can be added to desserts and pastries. The leaves also enhance cheese dishes.

Like the leaves, the dried root has a similar licorice-like taste, but it is a little earthier. Grind the dried roots into a powder to use in breads, cakes, muffins, or cookies. The seeds can also be used in cakes. The young, green stalks can be chopped and used to sweeten desserts. In the past it was quite popular to candy the stalks and use them to decorate cakes. One of the classics from England that my grandmother used to make is stewed rhubarb with angelica. The sweet taste of angelica offsets the tartness of the rhubarb.

TRADITIONAL RHUBARB AND ANGELICA

2 cups rhubarb stalks, sliced into ½-inch pieces

¼ cup angelica stems, finely chopped

⅓ cup sugar

2–4 tablespoons water

Toss the rhubarb and angelica with the sugar until they are coated. Add the water and simmer for about 10 minutes until the rhubarb is tender. This can be used as a pie filling, or it can be served as a stand-alone dessert or as a topping for ice cream or cheesecake.

....

How to Use the Essential Oils

Two oils are made from angelica. The oil from the roots ranges from colorless to pale yellow and turns yellow-brown with age. It has a rich, herbaceous, earthy scent. The oil from the seeds is colorless and has a herbaceous, earthy scent with a spicy undertone.

Massaging with either of the angelica essential oils (diluted in a carrier oil) eases the pain of arthritis and rheumatism and improves blood circulation. Angelica can be used on its own or blended with other essential oils. The following massage blend can be used to make bath salts for a soothing soak, too.

Angelica Warming Relief Massage Oil

5 drops angelica seed or root essential oil

4 drops rosemary essential oil

3 drops lemon balm essential oil

1 ounce carrier oil

Mix the essential oils together and then combine with the carrier oil.

....

Angelica is calming and soothing, and it helps to relieve anxiety, nervous tension, headache, and stress. Use it on its own in a diffuser or mix it in equal amounts with lavender and lemon balm. The combination of these three oils also makes a nice massage oil.

For skin care, angelica is effective for treating psoriasis. Mix one drop each of angelica seed and lemon balm essential oils with one teaspoon of apricot kernel or jojoba carrier oil. Gently dab the mixture on the affected areas. Angelica also helps brighten dull complexions. Combine the seed oil with lavender to make a cream that will soften and smooth the skin.

ANGELICA COMPLEXION CARE CREAM

½ cup shea butter

2–3 beeswax pastilles (pellets)

½ cup sweet almond carrier oil

1 cup distilled or filtered water

1 teaspoon angelica seed essential oil

1 teaspoon lavender essential oil

Combine the shea butter and beeswax in a jar and warm over low heat. When they begin to melt, add the carrier oil and stir gently. After everything melts, remove from heat and stir. Let it cool slightly, pour into a blender, and add the water and essential oils. Whip to get a light, creamy consistency. You may need to experiment with the amount of oils to get a consistency you like. Transfer the cream to a jar, allow it to cool, and then store.

Anise

(Pimpinella anisum L., syn. Anisum officinalis, Anisum vulgare)

Also known as: Aniseed, Sweet Cumin

Anise has been cultivated in Egypt for approximately four thousand years.[10] Its common name comes from the Latin *anisun*, which was derived from the Arab name for the plant *anysum*.[11] Both the Greeks and Romans used anise to flavor after-dinner cakes that also served as a digestive aid following huge banquets. Dioscorides, Hippocrates, and Pliny wrote about this herb and recommended it for various ailments. Anise was a highly-prized commodity to the Romans, who actually used the seeds to pay their taxes.

During the Middle Ages, its cultivation spread to Central Europe, where anise was used as a seasoning in a variety of dishes as well as a remedy for a wide range of complaints. As in ancient times, it was used as an after-dinner desert to help with digestion as well as a simple way to sweeten the breath. In England, the use of anise was so highly valued that King Edward I placed a tax on its import in 1305 to help pay for the repair of London Bridge.[12] Despite the tax, it remained popular, and by the mid-sixteenth century it was being cultivated in the British Isles.

As in times past, anise is used to flavor a wide variety of liqueurs including Benedictine, Chartreuse, ouzo, and of course, anisette. It should not be confused with star anise (*Illicium verum*). Anise is a cousin to caraway, dill, and fennel.

Medicinal Uses

Appetite stimulant, asthma, bad breath, bloating, breastfeeding problems, bronchitis, chest congestion, colds, cough, expectorant, flatulence, head lice, indigestion, menopausal discomforts, menstrual cramps, menstrual cycle problems, nasal congestion, postnatal depression, scabies, sleep aid, stomachache or pain, stress, upset stomach

Precautions and Contraindications

The herb: Avoid during pregnancy; should not be used by anyone with a condition that may worsen by exposure to estrogen.

---

10. Andrew Chevallier, *The Encyclopedia of Medicinal Plants: A Practical Reference Guide to Over 550 Key Herbs and Their Medicinal Uses* (New York: Doling Kindersley, 1996), 247.

11. Christopher Cumo, *Encyclopedia of Cultivated Plants: From Acacia to Zinnia, Vol. 1* (Santa Barbara, CA: ABC-CLIO, 2013), 27.

12. Michael Castleman, *The Healing Herbs: The Ultimate Guide to the Curative Power of Nature's Medicines* (New York, Bantam Books, 1995), 73.

The essential oils: Herbal precautions also apply; may cause skin irritation or dermatitis in some; use in moderation.

Parts of Plant Used

Herbal remedies: Seeds and leaves

Essential oils: Seeds

Culinary purposes: Seeds, leaves, and stalks

Growing and Harvesting

Only reaching about two feet tall, anise looks like a small, spindly version of Queen Anne's lace. Its lower leaves are rounded and coarsely toothed; the upper leaves are feathery. Umbels of delicate yellowish-white flowers grow at the tops of round, grooved stems. They bloom throughout the summer. The ribbed, flat seeds are gray-brown and oval. The seeds are approximately ⅛ inch long.

Type	Zone	Light	Soil	Moisture	Height	Spacing
Annual	Any	Full sun	Sandy loam	Dry	24"	12–18"

Plant anise where you want it to stay because it is difficult to transplant due to its long taproot. Its soil preference is often noted as "light and lean," meaning it likes sandy soil without compost or fertilizer. It likes a weed-free home, too. Anise is a good companion to coriander / cilantro and cabbage, but keep it away from carrots as it has a negative effect on them. Anise repels cabbage loopers and imported cabbage moths. Propagate this plant by sowing fresh seeds or let it help you as it readily reseeds.

Harvest leaves before the plant blooms. They can be screen dried or frozen. Cut off the seed heads and hang them in ventilated bags to catch the seeds.

How to Use the Herb

Spicy sweet and licorice-like, anise may be a familiar taste in commercial cough syrups and lozenges, however, this herb can do more than add flavor. A tea made with the seeds or a strong infusion of leaves can ease coughs, relieve bronchitis, and act as an expectorant.

ANISE TEA

1–1½ teaspoons seeds, crushed

1 cup boiling water

Combine the seeds and water. Steep for 15 to 20 minutes and strain.

Drink a cup of anise tea in the morning and one at night to break up congestion in the chest due to bronchitis and colds. This tea also helps ease asthma. A variation of it can be made with equal amounts of anise seeds and bay leaves. Of course, you could make your own cough syrup, too. The usual dose for syrup is one teaspoon as needed.

Anise Cough Syrup

1½–2 tablespoons anise seeds, crushed

2 tablespoons dried lemon balm leaves, crumbled

½ cup honey

1 quart water

Combine herbs and water in a saucepan and bring to a simmer. Keep on low heat until volume is reduced to a little less than half. Strain, return the liquid to the saucepan, and add the honey. Warm on low heat, stirring until the mixture is smooth. Let it cool a little and then pour into a jar. Store in the fridge where it will keep for several weeks.

With estrogen-like properties, anise is helpful during breastfeeding if insufficient milk is a problem. It also helps to ease postnatal depression. Make the plain anise tea as noted above and drink up to three cups a day. Anise tea also promotes menstrual flow and soothes menstrual cramps. For easing cramps, make a variation of the tea with equal amounts of anise, lemon balm, and marjoram. To ease hot flashes and other menopausal discomforts, make a mild tea with 1 teaspoon of crushed seeds in 1 cup of boiling water, and steep for ten to fifteen minutes.

Anise is an effective aid to soothe indigestion, prevent flatulence, and reduce bloating. It also stimulates the appetite. Make anise tea with 1½ to 2 teaspoons of crushed seeds in a cup of boiling water, and steep for ten to fifteen minutes. For a variation, make the tea with equal parts of anise seeds and chamomile. For stomachache or upset stomach, combine anise with peppermint and/or lemon balm.

Soothe the Tummy Anise Tea

½ teaspoon anise seeds, crushed

½ teaspoon dried peppermint leaves, crumbled

½ teaspoon dried lemon balm leaves, crumbled

1 cup boiling water

Combine the herbs and add the water. Steep for 20 minutes and strain. As an alternative, make a tincture and take ½ teaspoon up to 3 times a day.

To get rid of bad breath, boil a teaspoon of anise seeds for a few minutes, strain, and use as a mouthwash. Chewing on a few seeds will also sweeten the breath.

Both the leaves and seeds add unique flavor to a wide range of foods. Fresh, dried, or frozen leaves and stalks can be added to a range of foods. They can be roasted or sautéed for fish, poultry, and veggie dishes or added to curries and tomato sauces. The seeds intensify the sweetness of cakes and pastries. Add a pinch of crushed or powdered seeds to cookies, biscuits, or other baked goods. The seeds are also used with eggs, fruit, and cheese, and they are especially good in spinach and carrot dishes. Anise can be combined with cinnamon in sweet dishes and with bay for soups or stews.

For help in falling asleep, heat a cup of milk just below the boiling point, and then pour it over 1 teaspoon of crushed anise seeds. Let it steep until it is at a comfortably warm, drinkable temperature. Strain it, add a little honey, and let your cares melt away.

How to Use the Essential Oils

Anise seed essential oil has a spicy sweet and licorice-like scent. It is pale yellow in color. It provides another way to ease coughs, colds, and congestion by using it for a steam inhalation to help open sinus and bronchial airways. Just swish 4 drops of the oil into 1 quart of steaming water. As an alternative, blend it with peppermint and use 2 drops of each. Another option is to combine these two essential oils in a diffuser and place it in the sickroom. Also for the diffuser, mix equal parts of anise, lavender, and lemon balm for a blend that will reduce stress and promote restful sleep.

Anise is a mild antiparasitic and the essential oil can be used to treat head lice and scabies. For head lice, mix it with a carrier oil and work into the scalp. Because anise needs to be well diluted, use a 1 percent dilution ratio of 3 to 4 drops in 1 tablespoon of carrier oil. For scabies, an ointment works well. For this application, anise can be teamed up with other essential oils for added effectiveness and scent. Refer to appendix A for additional herbs that are used to treat scabies.

Anise Scabies Ointment

¼–½ cup jojoba or beeswax

½–1 cup carrier oil

1 teaspoon anise essential oil

1 teaspoon lavender, lemongrass, or peppermint essential oil

Place the jojoba or beeswax in a mason jar in a saucepan of water. Warm over low heat until it begins to melt; add the carrier oil. Stir gently for about 15 minutes. Remove from heat, add the essential oils, and stir. Test the thickness by placing a little on a plate and letting it cool in the fridge for a minute or two. If you want it firmer, add more jojoba or beeswax. If it's too thick, add a tiny bit of oil. Let it cool and then store in a cool, dark place.

Basil

(Ocimum basilicum L.)

Also known as: Common Basil, French Basil, Genovese Basil, Sweet Basil

Basil's genus and species names come from ancient Greek meaning "aromatic" or "smell" and "kingly" or "royal," respectively.[13] In later centuries, the French called it *Herbe Royale*. Basil is thought to have come from the plant known as Holy Basil (*Ocimum sanctum*) in India and transported into Greece by Alexander the Great.

This herb was used for medicinal and culinary purposes by the ancient Egyptians, Greeks, and Romans. Greek physician Dioscorides made note of it in his writing. Roman author Virgil also mentioned it. By the early sixteenth century, basil was being grown in northern Europe and England. During the Middle Ages it was used as a strewing herb, scattered on floors to freshen and clear the air. By the late sixteenth century, the Spanish had transported basil to North America.

Medicinal Uses

Abdominal pain, anxiety, asthma, bad breath, bronchitis, chronic fatigue, colds, cough, digestive system support, earache, fainting, flatulence, flu, gingivitis, hair care, hay fever, headaches, indigestion, infection, insect bites and stings, insect repellent, insomnia, motion sickness, mouth ulcers, muscle ache and pain, nasal congestion, nausea, nervous system support, sinusitis, stomachache or pain, stress, warts

Precautions and Contraindications

The herb: Therapeutic doses should be avoided during pregnancy and while nursing.

The essential oils: Avoid during pregnancy; use in moderation; may cause skin sensitization in some.

Parts of Plant Used

Herbal remedies: Leaves

Essential oils: Leaves and flowering tops

Culinary purposes: Leaves

Growing and Harvesting

Basil is a bushy plant that reaches one to two feet tall. Its oval leaves have prominent veins and a distinctive downward curl. They are yellow-green to dark green and very fragrant. White, pink, or purple flowers grow at the tops of stems and bloom from midsummer to autumn.

---

13. Rosemary Gladstar, *Medicinal Herbs: A Beginner's Guide* (North Adams, MA: Storey Publishing, 2012), 53.

Type	Zone	Light	Soil	Moisture	Height	Spacing
Annual	Any	Full sun	Loam	Moist	1–2'	12–18"

With a strong, spicy aroma, it is probably no surprise that basil is one of the most popular herbs in modern gardens. Basil is easily grown from seed, which is the method for propagation. While it prefers full sun, basil will tolerate partial shade. No matter where you grow it, keep it well composted. Basil repels asparagus beetles, fleas, flies, and mosquitoes. It is a good companion to peppers and tomatoes. Basil grows well in a container and makes an excellent house plant. Give it a sunny spot and water it when the surface of the soil begins to dry.

Leaves can be harvested throughout the season once the plant reaches eight inches in height and before the flowers bloom. Take the top leaves, which will encourage the plant to become bushy. Cut off flower spikes when they form for a longer harvest of leaves. The whole plant can be cut back to encourage new growth.

The leaves can be dried on screens but taste better when frozen. Blanch them before freezing by plunging them into boiling water for a few seconds until they wilt. Remove the leaves from the boiling water and then plunge them into a bowl of ice water to stop the wilting. This will help maintain their color and taste. Let the leaves dry and then store them in a container in the freezer. As an alternative, blend fresh leaves into a paste with olive oil before freezing.

How to Use the Herb

There are many types of basil, however, not all of them are used medicinally. The information in this book pertains to *Ocimum basilicum* only.

Perhaps best known for its flavor in pesto and tomato sauce, basil seems to go with just about anything. It has a spicy sweet flavor with a slight undertone of pepper that goes especially well with fish, poultry, cheese, eggs, vegetables, salads, and, of course, pasta. Basil blends well with garlic and thyme, and it makes a good infused cooking oil with them or on its own. Also tasty is a basil vinegar made with white vinegar.

The following is my simple pesto recipe. I like to tinker with it from time to time, adding different amounts or types of cheese or nuts, garlic, or even a dash of cayenne.

SIMPLY BASIL PESTO

4 cups fresh basil leaves, coarsely chopped

4 tablespoons pine nuts

½ cup olive oil

½ cup Parmesan cheese

Place the basil and nuts in a food processor or blender and pulse until it becomes a chunky paste. Add the olive oil and Parmesan in small amounts and sample as you go for taste and texture.

....

When basil leaves are fresh from the garden, who can resist cooking with them? In fact, eating more basil in late summer and early fall can help fend off colds, coughs, and the flu. Instead of adding it to food, drink a cup of basil tea several times a week. Basil can also help get hay fever under control.

When illness does strike, drinking basil tea will help fight infection. It relieves bronchitis, soothes coughs, and helps calm asthma attacks. A basil steam inhalation eases nasal congestion and sinusitis. The tea also soothes mouth ulcers, fights gingivitis, and gets rid of bad breath. Basil works well on its own for these purposes or it can be combined with peppermint for an added medicinal and flavor boost. On its own, a tea made with 2 teaspoons of basil can be used to make a warm compress to decrease the discomfort of an earache.

BASIL AND MINT INFECTION-FIGHTER TEA

1 teaspoon dried basil leaves, crumbled

1 teaspoon dried peppermint leaves, crumbled

1 cup boiling water

Combine the herbs and add the water. Steep for 10 to 15 minutes and strain.

....

Eating basil provides support for the digestive system, and when things get a little out of kilter, it can help put things right. A cup of basil tea after dinner relieves indigestion and flatulence. The tea also eases abdominal and stomach pain and reduces nausea. If you suffer from motion sickness, make a mild tea and take it along with you. Use 1 teaspoon of dried leaves in 1 cup of boiling water. Let it steep for ten minutes and then strain. Keep it warm in a thermos or drink it cool.

Basil has mild sedative properties that ease anxiety, headaches, insomnia, and stress. It also helps deal with chronic fatigue and is considered a tonic that supports the nervous system. For added effectiveness with these issues, combine basil with chamomile and lemon balm in a tea or infusion.

SOOTHE AND RELAX ME BASIL TEA

1 teaspoon dried basil leaves, crumbled

½ teaspoon dried lemon balm leaves, crumbled

½ teaspoon dried chamomile flowers, crumbled

1 cup boiling water

Combine the herbs and add the water. Steep for 10 to 20 minutes and strain.

....

Basil comes to the rescue for treating insect bites and stings by relieving the swelling and itching. It is especially soothing for wasp stings and mosquito bites. Make a poultice of fresh leaves or add water to dried leaves to make a paste. Apply to the affected area and use an adhesive bandage to hold the poultice in place. You can start treating bites and stings before going indoors by crushing and rubbing a basil leaf onto the affected area. In addition, crushed basil leaves rubbed on the skin work as an insect repellent. A basil poultice can also be used to treat warts. Hold it in place with an adhesive bandage until it cools. Repeat every day for five to seven days.

How to Use the Essential Oils

The essential oil made from basil ranges from colorless to pale yellow. Its scent is herbaceous and spicy sweet.

Basil essential oil relieves muscle aches and pains, especially after overexertion. It works well on its own, or it can be combined with lavender and marjoram for an aromatic treat that is equally soothing.

BASIL MUSCLE SOOTHING OIL

5 drops basil essential oil

5 drops lavender essential oil

3 drops marjoram essential oil

1 ounce carrier oil

Mix the essential oils together and then combine with the carrier oil.

....

Along with rosemary, basil can be used as a scalp treatment to stimulate hair growth. Use 1 drop of each essential oil in 1 teaspoon of carrier oil. Massage it into the scalp at bedtime, leave it on overnight, and then shampoo in the morning. Continue using the preparation until new growth begins. Basil essential oil is also effective to revive someone who has fainted.

Bay

(Laurus nobilis L.)

Also known as: Bay Laurel, Bay Tree, Roman Laurel, Sweet Bay, True Laurel

This plant's scientific name comes from the Latin *laurus*, meaning "to praise" or "to honor," and *nobilis*, "renowned." [14] It was customary for the ancient Greeks and Romans to praise people of accomplishment with crowns of bay laurel. In addition to decorating shrines and other public spaces with bay, the Greeks and Romans used the leaves for culinary and medicinal purposes. Dioscorides recommended bay to soothe the stomach, and Pliny said to use it to ease rheumatism. The leaves were also used as an insect repellent.

Hildegard of Bingen recommended bay for a range of ailments, as did herbalist Nicholas Culpeper several centuries later. During the Middles Ages, bay was used as a strewing herb for its fragrance and antiseptic properties. As a medicinal, bay was thought to prevent the plague.

Medicinal Uses

Appetite stimulant, arthritis, asthma, athlete's foot, bloating, bronchitis, bruises, carpal tunnel, colds, dandruff, digestive system support, flatulence, flu, hair care, indigestion, insect bites, insect repellent, jock itch, joint stiffness, muscle aches and pains, nasal congestion, rashes, rheumatism, scabies, sciatica, skin care, sore throat, sprains, tooth decay, vaginal yeast infection (vaginitis)

Precautions and Contraindications

The herb: Do not use bay when taking pain or sedative medications; avoid during pregnancy and when nursing.

The essential oils: Herbal precautions also apply; may cause sensitization or dermal irritation in some; use in moderation.

Parts of Plant Used

Herbal remedies: Leaves

Essential oils: Leaves and branchlets

Culinary purposes: Leaves

Growing and Harvesting

Bay may be more familiar as a small potted tree that is often cut into pom-poms or other topiary shapes. It is an evergreen tree that can grow up to fifty feet tall but it is most often kept pruned as a shrub. The dark green, leathery leaves are oval and sharply pointed. They grow on short stems. The

---

14. Roberta Wilson, *Aromatherapy* (New York: Penguin Putnam, 2002), 84.

small, greenish-yellow flowers grow in inconspicuous clusters and bloom in early spring. The oval berries are small and turn blue-black when they ripen.

Type	Zone	Light	Soil	Moisture	Height	Spacing
Perennial	8	Full sun to partial shade	Sandy loam	Moderately dry	2–50'	Depends on pruning

Bay is a lovely tree for a garden if you live in the right hardiness zones. Luckily, it grows well in a container, so those of us in the north can enjoy it, too. It works well as a houseplant because it is a slow grower that takes several years to reach two feet in height. Let the soil dry between waterings. Bay can be propagated with cuttings. It repels weevils.

Leaves can be harvested throughout the year, just cut off individual, older ones. Remove the stems and place the leaves on a screen with something on top so they dry flat. Turn them over every other day so they dry evenly. Bay leaves usually take about fifteen days to dry.

How to Use the Herb

Best known for its spicy aroma and subtle, earthy flavor, bay gives depth to soups, stews, marinades, and sauces. Add a leaf to the water when cooking grains or beans or making stock. Rub chicken with fresh leaves before roasting or tuck a leaf into a slit in a potato so it bakes with the flavor and aroma of bay. In addition, a couple of dried leaves in the flour canister serve to repel any insect invaders.

Bay is part of the traditional *herbes de Provence* blend along with fennel, rosemary, and thyme. Not only does bay coax out the flavor of food and other herbs, it also supports the digestive system. Bay improves the absorption of nutrients and aids in breaking down heavy food, especially meat. A tea made with fresh bay leaves comes to the rescue to soothe indigestion, bloating, and flatulence. It also stimulates the appetite. Fresh leaves are not as strong in aroma or flavor as dried ones.

The combination of bay's antiseptic, anti-inflammatory, antifungal, and antibacterial properties make it a good choice for a wide range of topical applications. Brew a strong tea for a foot soak or sitz bath to relieve the itching and inflammation of athlete's foot, jock itch, and vaginal yeast infections. As an alternative, use equal amounts of bay and lavender. Drinking it as a tea and using it topically can help heal from both inside and out. Alternatively, infuse an oil to make an ointment, which may be easier for topical application.

BAY AND LAVENDER HEALING TEA

1–2 teaspoons fresh bay leaves, crumbled

1–2 teaspoons fresh lavender flowers, crumbled

1 cup boiling water

Combine the herbs and add the water. Steep for 10 to 20 minutes and strain.

Bay is also effective for healing bruises and rashes. An infusion or strong tea can be used for a compress to place on the affected area. A poultice works well, too. For treating insect bites and scabies, combine bay with lemongrass in an infusion, which can be used straight or made into a cream.

Call on the warming and anti-inflammatory effects of bay by using an infused oil for massage. This oil also works well to relieve the pain and stiffness of rheumatism and arthritis. In addition, it eases muscle aches, sprains, sciatica, carpal tunnel, and joint stiffness. For a healing soak in the tub, combine bay with rosemary and lavender in an infusion to add to your bath water.

HEALING BAY MUSCLE SOAK INFUSION

3–4 tablespoons fresh rosemary leaves, crumbled

3–4 tablespoons fresh lavender flowers, crumbled

1 tablespoon fresh bay leaves, crumbled

per quart boiling water

Combine the herbs and then add the water. Steep for 30 to 45 minutes and strain.

....

As an aromatic with antiviral and antibacterial properties, bay is helpful for relieving cold and flu symptoms. A steam inhalation will soothe inflammation, ease nasal congestion, and help clear the respiratory airways. This helps to ease asthma and bronchitis as well. Combine bay with rosemary to make a chest rub. The physically warming effects and the aromatic vapors of these herbs work together to provide relief and healing.

BAY CHEST RUB INFUSION AND OINTMENT

Ingredients for the infused oil	*Ingredients for the ointment*
1 tablespoon dried bay leaves, crumbled	¼–½ cup beeswax or jojoba
1 tablespoon dried rosemary leaves, crumbled	1 cup infused oil
1 cup oil	

First, infuse an oil by combining it with the herbs in a double boiler. On very low heat, simmer for 45 to 60 minutes. Remove from heat and let cool. Use a stainless steel strainer lined with cheesecloth over a bowl to strain, and then fold the cheesecloth over the herbs to press out as much oil as possible.

To make the ointment, place the jojoba or beeswax in a mason jar in a saucepan of water. Warm over low heat until it begins to melt, then add the infused oil. Stir gently with a fork for about 15 minutes. Let it cool. Cover and store in a cool, dark place.

....

A bay infusion also makes a good gargle to soothe a sore throat. Used as a mouthwash, it helps fight tooth decay. Bay is also useful as a tonic for the hair and scalp, especially if dandruff is a problem. Make an infusion, let it cool to room temperature, and strain. After shampooing and rinsing your hair, pour the infusion over your head, and then massage it into your scalp. Wrap a towel around your head and leave the bay rinse on for fifteen to twenty minutes. Rinse thoroughly with water.

Bay is also good for the skin. An infusion can be used for a facial splash or to make a soothing cream. A little lavender can be added to the infusion to make it even more fragrant and healing.

How to Use the Essential Oils

Bay essential oil has a fresh, herbaceous, and slightly camphoraceous scent. Its color is greenish-yellow.

Just as an infusion can be used for a steam inhalation to relieve cold and flu symptoms, so too can the essential oil. Add five to ten drops to a quart of boiling water. The essential oil can also be used as a nasal inhaler that you can take with you wherever you go. For double power, use thyme to make a breathing blend. (Be sure to read the essential oil information and precautions in the profile on thyme.) Without touching the bottle to your nose, take a couple of deep inhalations, put the cap on the bottle, and set it aside. Repeat in half an hour to an hour or as needed.

BAY COLD RELIEF NASAL INHALER

2 drops bay essential oil

2 drops thyme essential oil

Combine the essential oils in a small, clean bottle.

Borage

(Borago officinalis L.)

Also known as: Bee Bread, Bugloss, Burrage, Star Flower

Borage flowers attract bees and yield a rich honey, which is the source of its name Bee Bread. In addition to medicinal purposes, the Greeks used borage to flavor wine. Greek physician Dioscorides noted that this herb brought about a sense of well-being. Pliny called the plant *Euphrosinum* because it was said to bring happiness.[15] Centuries later, herbalist John Gerard recommended it for the relief of melancholy. Borage was considered an herb to "comfort the heart" and relieve sorrow.[16]

The Roman legions introduced borage into northern Europe and the British Isles. Both Roman and Celtic warriors used borage before battles because it was said to bolster courage and strength. "Borage for courage" was a belief held for over a thousand years up to the time of the Crusades when knights mixed it in their wine to boost their bravery. Of course, there is much speculation that their courage may have come more from the wine than from borage. Nevertheless, this plant was also used medicinally and medieval herbalists prescribed it for a range of ailments.

Medicinal Uses

Acne, bladder inflammation, boils, bronchitis, catarrh, chest congestion, chronic fatigue, colds, cough, dermatitis, eczema, expectorant, fever, menopausal discomforts, premenstrual syndrome (PMS), psoriasis, rashes, Raynaud's disease, rheumatoid arthritis, skin care, stress, stretch marks, temporomandibular joint pain (TMJ)

Precautions and Contraindications

The herb: Avoid during pregnancy or when nursing; those with liver disease should avoid its use.

The carrier oil: Herbal precautions also apply.

Parts of Plant Used

Herbal remedies: Leaves and flowers

Carrier oil: Seeds

Culinary purposes: Leaves, flowers, and stems

---

15. Ann Bonar, *Herbs: A Complete Guide to the Cultivation and Use of Wild and Domesticated Herbs* (New York, MacMillan Publishing, 1985), 50.

16. Edith Grey Wheelwright, *Medicinal Plants and Their History* (New York: Dover Publications, 1974), 148.

Growing and Harvesting

The hallmark of borage is its intensely blue, star-shaped flowers that grow in drooping clusters. They bloom mid to late summer. The gray-green, oval leaves are pointed and have prominent veins. The hollow, upright stems have many leafy branches. Both the stems and leaves are covered with tiny hairs. Borage grows between one and three feet tall. Its sprawling branches give the plant a rounded shape.

Type	Zone	Light	Soil	Moisture	Height	Spacing
Annual	Any	Full sun	Sandy or chalky loam	Moist	1–3'	24"

Borage tolerates partial shade in southern regions and it is sometimes a biennial lasting two seasons. This plant grows well in a container located in a sunny spot. Borage can be propagated by sowing fresh seeds or let the plant do it for you as it readily self-seeds. This herb is a companion to beans, cucumbers, strawberries, and tomatoes. It repels tomato hornworms, and as mentioned, bees love borage. Honey bees are especially attracted to it.

Leaves can be harvested any time, and harvest flowers when they are fully open. Just snip off individual leaves and flowers or flower clusters.

How to Use the Herb

Borage is a symbol of summer, which is the time to take advantage of using it as it does not dry or freeze well for long-term storage. The flavor and potency fades as the leaves and flowers dry out.

Summer colds and illness can be frustrating because it is difficult to stay indoors when the weather is warm and sunny. Take advantage of having borage in your garden. Its mild expectorant properties will help clear chest congestion and relieve bronchitis and other coughs as well as catarrh. Drink three cups a day of the Borage Summer Cough Relief Infusion.

BORAGE SUMMER COUGH RELIEF INFUSION

6–8 tablespoons fresh leaves and/or flowers, chopped

1 quart boiling water

Pour the water over the chopped herb. Steep for 30 to 60 minutes, and then strain. Store in the fridge.

For an extra boost and different taste, make the infusion with 6 tablespoons of borage and 2 tablespoons of peppermint. Also, an infusion using only borage flowers makes a good cough syrup. Combine ⅔ cup of infusion and ⅓ cup of honey in a saucepan. Stir over low heat until the honey becomes less viscous. Cool and store. Take a teaspoon several times a day or as needed.

To break a fever, simmer a handful of borage leaves and/or flowers in 1 pint of water for five minutes. Let it cool, strain, and then drink half a cup at a time over a three hour period.

Borage leaves have diuretic and anti-inflammatory properties, which help to ease bladder inflammation. Make a syrup of the leaves and take a tablespoon once a day, or make a tincture and take a teaspoon twice a day. A tincture of borage is a good way to ease stress, too. Take a teaspoon three times a day for two to three weeks. A tea of borage flowers and lemon balm also helps to combat stress as well as chronic fatigue. Additionally, the combination of borage and lemon balm eases the symptoms of PMS and menopausal discomforts.

BORAGE AND LEMON BALM TEA

2 teaspoons fresh borage flowers, chopped

2 teaspoons fresh lemon balm leaves, chopped

1 cup boiling water

Combine the herbs and then add the water. Steep for 10 to 15 minutes and strain.

....

Of course, just as borage carrier oil is good for treating skin problems, so too is the fresh plant. Make an infusion of leaves and/or flowers for a calming bath that will nourish your skin and heal any irritation. The infusion can also be used to make a cream to treat itchy skin or rashes. Use a poultice made from the leaves to treat and soothe boils.

Like other herbs, borage has many culinary uses. The flowers have a slight cucumber taste that goes well in green salads. Float a borage flower in a glass of white wine or sparkling water as a festive decoration that also adds a little flavor. Alternatively, freeze flowers in an ice cube tray (one in each section) for icing summer drinks. Float borage flowers in a fruit punch or add a few leaves to a pitcher of lemonade to add color and flavor.

The leaves can be used like spinach either raw, steamed, or sautéed. The stems can be peeled, chopped, and used like celery. Leaves and/or stems can be added to fish, poultry, or vegetable dishes or used in salad dressings. The leaves and stems blend well with dill, mint, and garlic, and on their own they make a nice, lightly flavored vinegar. Also, start your summer mornings with a borage treat for your breakfast toast.

BREAKFAST BORAGE [17]

1 tablespoon fresh leaves, chopped

4 ounces cream cheese or cottage cheese

---

17. Bonar, *Herbs*, 50.

Stir in the borage leaves until they are evenly distributed throughout the cream cheese or cottage cheese. Spoon it onto toast or have it alongside.

....

How to Use the Carrier Oil

Borage oil is light yellow with a light, sweet scent. It lasts approximately six months in the refrigerator. Borage is often mixed with a lighter-textured oil such as sweet almond.

This oil is the skin's best friend. It contains a range of vitamins and minerals that heal the skin and encourages cell regeneration. It soothes the inflammation and irritation of acne, dermatitis, eczema, psoriasis, and rashes. Use a drop or two of the oil and gently massage it into the affected area or lightly dab it on. Massage the oil into the fingers for relief of Raynaud's disease or use it on the fingers and toes for rheumatoid arthritis pain. Also, massage the jaw to ease temporomandibular joint pain (TMJ).

Borage promotes healthy skin and is especially good for dry or mature skin. It also helps reduce some stretch marks. Lavender essential oil is included in the Borage and Lavender Skin Cream for additional healing power and to add fragrance.

Borage and Lavender Skin Cream

Ingredients for the infusion
2 tablespoons dried lavender leaves and
  flowers, crumbled
1 cup boiling water

Ingredients for the cream
½ cup shea butter
2–3 beeswax pastilles (pellets)
¼ cup borage oil
¼ cup almond or other light oil
1 cup lavender infusion

First, make a lavender infusion by steeping the dried lavender in the water for 40 to 50 minutes, and then strain.

To make the cream, combine the shea butter and beeswax in a jar and warm over low heat. When they begin to melt, add the oil and gently stir. After everything melts, remove from heat and stir. Let it cool slightly, pour into a blender, and add the lavender infusion. Whip to get a light, creamy consistency. You may need to vary the amount of oils to get a consistency you like. Transfer the cream to a jar, allow to cool, and store.

Caraway

(Carum carvi L.)

Also known as: Carum, Common Caraway, Roman Cumin

According to archeological evidence, the use of caraway dates back more than five thousand years.[18] Caraway was mentioned in the Egyptian Ebers papyrus and it was found in the tombs of the pharaohs. Its genus name comes from the Greek *karon*, meaning "annual or biennial herb."[19] *Carvi*, the Latin name for caraway, was noted by Roman naturalist Pliny as being named for the Caria region in Asia Minor.[20]

The Greeks and Romans used caraway for medicinal and culinary purposes. It was an important herb of commerce in the ancient world. In later centuries, caraway essential oil became a valuable commodity in Central Europe, especially Romania, which developed a reputation for producing exceptional medicinal herbs. While they were valued throughout Europe during the Middle Ages for medicinal purposes, the seeds became most popular for baking in Northern European countries. From Tudor to Victorian times in England, caraway was *the* seed in seed cake, which was a popular teatime treat.

Medicinal Uses

Acne, appetite stimulant, bad breath, belching, bloating, boils, breastfeeding problems, bronchitis, bruises, catarrh, cough, digestive system support, flatulence, indigestion, irritable bowel syndrome (IBS), laryngitis, menstrual cramps, nausea, postnatal depression, scabies, skin care, stomachache or pain, upset stomach

Precautions and Contraindications

The herb: Excessive amounts of seeds should not be eaten during pregnancy.

The essential oils: May cause skin irritation in some.

Parts of Plant Used

Herbal remedies: Seeds and leaves

Essential oils: Seeds

Culinary purposes: Seeds, leaves, and roots

---

18. Kowalchik, *Rodale's Illustrated Encyclopedia of Herbs*, 63.

19. Allen J. Coombes, *Dictionary of Plant Names* (Portland, OR: Timber Press, 1985), 48.

20. Marina Heilmeyer, *Ancient Herbs* (Los Angeles, CA: Getty Publications, 2007), 30.

Growing and Harvesting

Caraway has slender stems that are ridged and hollow. Its light green, feathery leaves are similar to carrot leaves. Tiny white flowers grow in umbel clusters and bloom during the late summer. The root looks like a parsnip. The slightly crescent-shaped seeds are ridged and pointed at both ends. Caraway reaches eighteen to twenty-four inches tall and resembles Queen Anne's lace. It is closely related to anise, dill, and fennel.

Type	Zone	Light	Soil	Moisture	Height	Spacing
Biennial	3	Full sun	Sandy loam	Slightly dry	18–24"	6–8"

Caraway is a little quirky. Although it is a biennial, it sometimes goes to seed in the first year. However, it may continue growing through the second season and set seed in the third. In its first year, the plant may not even reach twelve inches tall. Caraway prefers full sun but will tolerate partial shade in southern areas. It is a good companion to peas but does not like to grow near fennel. Propagate this herb by sowing fresh seeds or let it help you as it readily reseeds.

Leaves can be harvested in the first and second seasons and screen dried. When seed heads begin to ripen, enclose them in paper bags or cut the entire stem to hang dry. The roots can be dug up after the seeds have been harvested.

How to Use the Herb

Caraway is most widely known for aiding digestion. While the leaves and roots help the digestive system handle starchy foods, the seeds are a powerhouse when it comes to treating problems. For indigestion or upset stomach, munch on a teaspoonful of seeds a few at a time, or make a tea with 2 teaspoons of crushed seeds. Also, eating just a few seeds will help get rid of bad breath. Caraway's antispasmodic properties ease stomach pain and aid in dealing with IBS. Combine it with peppermint and lemon balm for tasty relief. Take a couple of tablespoons of the tea at intervals until the pain subsides.

CARAWAY TUMMY TROUBLE TEA

1 teaspoon caraway seeds, crushed

½ teaspoon dried peppermint leaves, crumbled

½ teaspoon dried lemon balm leaves, crumbled

1 cup boiling water

Combine the herbs and add the water. Steep for 10 to 20 minutes and strain.

For belching, bloating, or flatulence, make a tea with just 1 teaspoon of crushed seeds. This tea also eases nausea. To stimulate a poor appetite, take a teaspoon of caraway tincture three times a day.

Caraway is a tonic for the digestive system and a treat for the taste buds. The fact that every part of the plant is edible makes it easy to add to the diet. The taste of the seeds has been described as a combination of anise and dill. They are spicy with a slight peppery undertone. The seeds can be mixed with savory or sweet foods, and are most famous for adding flavor to breads and cakes. They can be used whole or crushed in egg dishes, with cheese, and a wide range of veggies and meats. The leaves have a milder flavor, more like dill, and can be used fresh in soups, stews, and fruit or vegetable salads. Not only do the roots look like parsnips, they can be cooked and eaten like them, too. After harvesting autumn vegetables and roots, enjoy the flavors and beauty of the season by roasting them together on a chilly evening.

Autumn Veggie Root Roast with Caraway

Red potatoes, unpeeled, cut into 1-inch pieces

Carrots, peeled, cut into 1-inch pieces

Butternut squash, peeled, cut into 1-inch pieces

Caraway root, peeled, cut into 1-inch pieces

Onion, peeled, quartered lengthwise

Olive oil

Rosemary and/or thyme

Garlic cloves, peeled and chopped

Apple, grated

Maple syrup

The amounts and exactly which vegetables are a matter of personal taste. Preheat the oven to 400° Fahrenheit. In a large bowl, combine the potatoes, carrots, squash, caraway, and onion. Drizzle with olive oil and toss so they are completely coated. Add the rosemary and/or thyme and toss again. Move the veggies to a large pan and roast for 30 minutes, stirring about every 10 minutes. Add the garlic, stir, and return to the oven for 20 minutes. Stir and then sprinkle the grated apple over the vegetables and drizzle with a little maple syrup. Roast for another 10 or 15 minutes or until the vegetables are fork-tender.

Caraway is a warming and relaxing herb that relieves menstrual cramps and increases the flow of breast milk. It also helps to ease postnatal depression. Before crushing the seeds for making any preparation, toast them in a dry frying pan just long enough to bring out their aroma and enhance their flavor.

SIMPLY CARAWAY TEA

1–2 teaspoons seeds, crushed

1 cup boiling water

Combine the herbs and add the water. Steep for 10 to 15 minutes and strain.

....

For menstrual cramps, drink two or three cups of the tea a day. Drink one cup a day when breastfeeding. In addition, the tea can be made with equal amounts of caraway and fennel seeds.

How to Use the Essential Oils

Caraway essential oil ranges from colorless to pale yellow, to yellowish-brown. It has a warm, sweet-spicy scent.

A steam inhalation with caraway oil is helpful for treating bronchitis, coughs, laryngitis, and catarrh. Just swish 4 drops of oil into 1 quart of steaming water. Or, you can blend it with basil using 2 drops of each. In addition, place a few drops of caraway essential oil in a clean bottle to use as a nasal inhaler to take with you on the go. Without touching the bottle to your nose, take a couple of deep inhalations. Repeat in a half hour to an hour or as needed.

A facial steam with caraway stimulates the skin and improves the complexion. Use the essential oil to make a topical ointment for skin problems such as acne and boils. The ointment is effective for treating bruises and scabies also. Combine it with lavender for a boost in effectiveness and a wonderful fragrance.

FRAGRANT HEALING CARAWAY OINTMENT

¼–½ cup jojoba or beeswax

½–1 cup coconut or other carrier oil

1 teaspoon caraway essential oil

1 teaspoon lavender essential oil

Place the jojoba or beeswax in a mason jar in a saucepan of water. Warm over low heat until it begins to melt; add the carrier oil. Stir gently for about 15 minutes. Remove from heat, add the essential oils and stir. Test the thickness by placing a little on a plate and letting it cool in the fridge for a minute or two. If you want it firmer, add more jojoba or beeswax. If it's too thick, add a tiny bit of oil. Let it cool, and then store in a cool, dark place.

Cayenne
(Capsicum annuum L.)

Also known as: Bird Pepper, Capsicum, Cayenne Pepper, Chili Pepper, Red Chilies

The genus name *Capsicum* comes from the Greek *kapto*, which means "to bite." [21] This is apropos for an herb that has real bite. Even though it was cultivated in South America, India, and Africa for thousands of years, it wasn't until historian Peter Martyr (1457–1526) wrote an account of Christopher Columbus's "discoveries" that cayenne caught the attention of Europeans. By the mid-sixteenth century, it had become established in European cooking and herbal medicine.

In modern times, cayenne has been used to add extra zing to ginger ale. Although cayenne is not related to the familiar black pepper, it was so named because it is pungent like black pepper. While it may seem odd, this fiery pepper is soothing and restorative. Paprika and Tabasco sauce are made from other varieties of *capsicum* peppers.

Medicinal Uses
Arthritis, bloating, cardiovascular system support, carpal tunnel, chest congestion, chilblains, chills, cholesterol, colds, cuts and scrapes, digestive system support, fibromyalgia, flatulence, flu, hangover, headache, immune system support, joint stiffness, migraine, muscle aches and pains, nasal congestion, nerve pain, rheumatoid arthritis, shingles, sore throat

Precautions and Contraindications
The herb: Use in small amounts; excessive internal use may cause upset stomach; those with irritable bowel syndrome (IBS) or chronic bowel inflammation should avoid the internal use of cayenne; may aggravate acidity and heartburn; may increase hot flashes during menopause.

The essential oils: Avoid during pregnancy.

When handling the peppers, wear gloves and be careful not to touch your eyes when working with cayenne. If you do, rinse with milk.

Parts of Plant Used
Herbal remedies: Peppers

Essential oils: Seeds

Culinary purposes: Peppers

---

21. Coombes, *Dictionary of Plant Names*, 47.

Growing and Harvesting

Reaching two to three feet in height, cayenne's angular branches give the plant a bushy appearance. Its broad, dark green leaves have an elliptical shape. Growing on long stems in drooping pairs or clusters, the five-petaled flowers are white to yellowish-white and may be tinged with purple. The pendulous fruits (peppers) are long and thin, and contain small, kidney-shaped, white seeds. The peppers are green, then turn various shades of red, orange, or yellow as they ripen. They have a pungent smell.

Type	Zone	Light	Soil	Moisture	Height	Spacing
Annual	7	Full sun	Any	Moist	24–36"	24"

The word *annuum* in its name indicates that it is an annual, but in southern zones the plant is a perennial. Because cayenne needs a long growing season, it is often a good plant to grow in a container in northern areas. During cooler weather keep it indoors and then move it outside for the summer once the temperature gets above sixty degrees Fahrenheit. Cayenne is an aid in the vegetable garden as it repels moths and weevils. It is a good companion to cucumbers, eggplants, and tomatoes. Plant peppermint near your cayenne to deter aphids. Cayenne is propagated by sowing fresh seeds.

Pick the chilies when they turn red, orange, or yellow in late summer or early fall. As mentioned above, it is a good idea to wear gloves as handling the fruit can burn the skin. Cut the stems instead of pulling the peppers off the branches to avoid damaging the fruit. Use a big sewing needle and thick thread to string the chilies through their tops, creating a chili pepper wreath. Hang it in a warm place. When the peppers are dry, use a food processor to grind them into a powder. Like the powder, the whole, dried chilies can be stored in airtight containers in a cool, dark place.

How to Use the Herb

Cayenne is a warming herb that aids poor circulation by stimulating blood flow. High in antioxidants, cayenne is beneficial for heart and cardiovascular health and it may help lower cholesterol. Try the following recipe for a heart-healthy drink.

Cayenne Heart and Head Tonic

8 ounces tomato juice (or V-8)

A drop or two of cayenne tincture (to taste)

Mix thoroughly before drinking.

A contributing factor to headaches, especially migraine, is blood vessel contraction in the brain. A pinch of powdered cayenne dissolved in hot water taken at the onset of a migraine may not completely eliminate the headache, but it will bring some relief. After taking this remedy, follow it with a little bit of milk to cool the mouth. Cayenne has become known as a head-clearing herb because it helps lift mental fog and relieves symptoms of hangover.

Cayenne's best-known head-clearing attribute is the relief of nasal congestion due to colds and flu. It clears congestion in the chest, too. The Cayenne Cold and Flu Tea can also be used as a gargle for sore throat, as can the above-mentioned migraine remedy.

Cayenne Cold and Flu Tea
1 pinch cayenne, powdered

1 teaspoon lemon juice

1 teaspoon honey

1 cup boiling water

In a mug, add the cayenne powder to the lemon juice. Pour in the water, and then stir in a spoonful of honey. Let it cool just enough to drink.

....

Cayenne is high in vitamins A and C and supports the immune system, which helps in preventing colds and flu. Think of using the heat of summer to warm your winter by adding cayenne to your diet when cold weather sets in. Include a little cayenne in pesto to add a little kick for winter months (see the profile on basil for a recipe), or try the Spicy Veggie Sprinkle. Another health and healing attribute of cayenne is that it strengthens the digestive system and is an aid to inefficient digestion. Boosting the metabolism, cayenne helps reduce flatulence and bloating.

Spicy Veggie Sprinkle with Cayenne [22]
2 tablespoons coriander, powdered

2 teaspoons cumin, powdered

¼ teaspoon cayenne, powdered

Combine ingredients and mix well. Sprinkle a little over warm vegetables before serving.

....

---

22. Kami McBride, *The Herbal Kitchen: 50 Easy-to-Find Herbs and Over 250 Recipes to Bring Lasting Health to Your Family* (San Francisco: Conari Press, 2010), 223.

Externally this herb can be used to relieve muscle aches and pains, joint stiffness, fibromyalgia, and chills. Rub cayenne-infused oil on arthritic joints, sore muscles, or the site of nerve pain. It is especially good for treating carpal tunnel pain and rheumatoid arthritis. Because cayenne is diluted in oil, it does not burn the skin. Cayenne warms and soothes by dilating small capillaries and increasing blood circulation. Use a little oil on small areas of skin and rub in well. Additionally, cayenne-infused oil can be used to treat shingles and chilblains but only if they are unbroken.

CAYENNE RUBBING OIL

1 teaspoon powdered cayenne

½ cup oil

Start with 1 teaspoon of pepper and mix well. Test on a small area of skin. If you don't feel any warming effects, increase the amount of cayenne by ½ teaspoon and test again. It is important to mix and test slowly to get the ratio that works best for you.

....

The rubbing oil can be used to make a cream or ointment, which may be easier to use for some applications. In addition, a liniment of cayenne is a good way to relieve muscle pain and joint stiffness.

Keep powdered cayenne on hand for first aid. While it helps increase the flow of blood when taken internally, on an open wound cayenne stops the bleeding. Just sprinkle a little of the powder on a cut. Yes, it will sting but only for a moment. Not only will it stop the pain but it will also disinfect the cut. Of course, seek medical attention if you have more than a superficial wound.

How to Use the Essential Oils

Cayenne essential oil is dark red with a strong, pungent, and spicy scent. It is not usually blended with other essential oils.

Instead of powdered cayenne, use the essential oil to make the Cayenne Rubbing Oil to relieve aches and pains. Start with 1 drop in 1 tablespoon of carrier oil. Like using the powder, test the oil on a small area of skin. If you don't feel any warming effects, increase the amount of cayenne by 1 drop and test again. This mixture can be rubbed on cold feet in the winter to enhance circulation. When suffering from a cold, dab a little of the essential oil on a tissue and waft it under your nose to open the sinuses.

The Chamomiles

German Chamomile *(Matricaria recutita L., syn. M. chamomilla)*

Also known as: Blue Chamomile, Hungarian Chamomile, Mayweed, Wild Chamomile

Roman Chamomile *(Chamaemelum nobile L., syn. Anthemis nobilis)*

Also known as: English Chamomile, Garden Chamomile, Maythen, Sweet Chamomile

Both plants also known as: Camomile, True Chamomile

Chamomile has been used medicinally for a range of ailments since the time of the ancient Egyptians. Greek physician Hippocrates included chamomile in his writings. This herb's name comes from the Greek *chamailmelon*, meaning "ground apple," which describes the scent of Roman chamomile.[23] Flavored with Roman chamomile, the name of the Spanish sherry Manzinilla means "little apple."[24]

Although German chamomile has been considered a weed at times, both herbs have medicinal properties and have been used interchangeably. Medieval monks deemed chamomile the "plants' physician" because of its healthy effect on other garden plants.[25] Chamomile was used throughout the Middle Ages as a strewing herb because stepping on the flowers releases their sweet fragrance. In addition, chamomile has been used to create various yellow dyes.

Medicinal Uses

Acne, arthritis, belching, bloating, breast problems, burns, colic, colitis, Crohn's disease, cuts and scrapes, dandruff, digestive system support, earache, eczema, eye problems, fever, gastritis, hair care, hay fever, headache, heartburn, indigestion, inflammation, insect bites and stings, insomnia, mastitis, muscle aches and pain, nausea, nervous tension, rashes, rheumatism, rheumatoid arthritis, skin care, sleep aid, sore throat, sprains, stomachache or pain, stress, sunburn, teething pain, toothache, upset stomach

Precautions and Contraindications

The herb: Although chamomile is an antiallergenic for most people, those who have allergies to plants in the *Asteraceae* family should check for sensitivity before using it; avoid ingesting when taking prescription blood thinners.

The essential oils: May cause dermatitis in some.

---

23. Wilson, *Aromatherapy*, 80.
24. Bonar, *Herbs*, 54.
25. Jack Staub, 75 *Exceptional Herbs for Your Garden* (Layton, UT: Gibbs Smith, 2008), 48.

Part of Plant Used

Herbal remedies, essential oils, and culinary purposes: Flowers

Growing and Harvesting

With branching stems, German chamomile stands erect and can reach two or three feet in height. Roman chamomile is a spreading herb with stems that creep along the ground. It is usually less than nine inches high. Both plants have small, daisy-like flowers with white petals and yellow centers that grow at the ends of the stems. German chamomile flowers are less fragrant than the apple-scented Roman. Both plants have feathery, downy leaves, however, Roman chamomile's leaves are slightly more coarse.

Herb	Type	Zone	Light	Soil	Moisture	Height	Spacing
German	Annual	Any	Full sun to partial shade	Sandy	Moderately dry	30"	6–8"
Roman	Perennial	5	Partial shade	Loam	Moderately moist	8–9"	18"

The seeds of German chamomile can be planted in the autumn or spring. Propagate it by sowing fresh seeds or let it help you as it readily reseeds. German chamomile produces more flowers than Roman. Even though Roman chamomile is easy to grow from seed, they are so tiny that they can be difficult to work with. When establishing plants in the garden, space them about eighteen inches apart to give the stems room to creep along the ground. While it is a hardy plant, in colder zones it's a good idea to mulch it over for the winter. Propagate Roman chamomile through cuttings or division of roots.

As mentioned, chamomile is the "plants' physician" helping to increase the vitality of other plants in the garden. It is especially beneficial for basil, dill, and peppermint. In the vegetable garden, German chamomile improves the growth and flavor of cabbages, cucumbers, and onions. Both chamomiles attract predatory wasps and a wide array of beneficial insects including hoverflies. Chamomile repels fleas.

The flowers of both chamomiles should be harvested just before they fully open. With German chamomile, cut the flower stems from the plant. Bundle them loosely and hang, or cut off the flowers and screen dry them. Because the stems of Roman chamomile are short, it is easier to just pinch the blossoms from the plant and screen dry. Handle flowers gently; however, any that are inadvertently damaged can be used for the following plant spray.

CHAMOMILE PROTECTIVE PLANT SPRAY

1 handful flowers

1 quart cold water

Soak the flowers for 2 or 3 days and then strain the liquid into a spray bottle. Mist plants in the garden to protect them against fungal disease and to revive plants that appear to be distressed. The spent chamomile flowers can go on the compost pile.

....

How to Use the Herb

First and foremost, chamomile is known as a pleasant, mild tea, which is its only culinary use. A medicinal-strength tea calms the stomach and nerves and aids in getting restful sleep as well as treating insomnia. In addition, it supports a healthy digestive system. Chamomile's antispasmodic properties help to relieve heartburn, belching, and stomachache. Drinking the tea regularly can aid in soothing colitis, gastritis, and Crohn's disease. In addition, chamomile tea taken by nursing mothers helps relieve colic in their babies.

PLAIN AND SIMPLE CHAMOMILE TEA

2 teaspoons dried flowers, crumbled

1 cup boiling water

Pour the water over the herb. Steep for at least 10 minutes and strain. Add a little honey to taste.

....

Combine chamomile with an equal amount of spearmint to make a tea for extra help in soothing an upset stomach or quelling nausea. For indigestion and bloating, make a tea with equal parts of chamomile and fennel seeds.

Chamomile tea is helpful during hay fever season to ease symptoms. In addition, the tea can be used as a gargle to soothe a sore throat. As an alternative to the tea, use 2 teaspoons of chamomile tincture in 1 cup of warm water.

Make a strong chamomile tea, let it cool, and use it to prepare a compress for headache relief. Dip a washcloth in the tea and then place it across the forehead from temple to temple. Taking a spoonful of chamomile honey can also bring relief. In addition to headaches, a cool chamomile compress can help bring down a fever, reduce inflammation, and ease sprains. A warm compress helps to soothe puffy, irritated eyes. To soothe sunburn, chill a jar of chamomile tea in the fridge and gently dab it on to cool and heal the skin.

For a relaxing soak in the bathtub, make a chamomile infusion. Fill a small muslin or cotton pouch with chamomile flowers while you boil a quart of water. Drop the pouch of flowers in the water, stir, and then put a lid on the pot. Let it steep for about thirty minutes. Run your bath water and then add the chamomile infusion. You can remove the pouch of flowers or let it continue releasing beneficial oils as you soak away your stress along with muscle aches and pains. Add a handful of rose petals for an extra aromatic treat. While you are in the tub, lean back and dip your head in the water or make a separate infusion for your hair. A chamomile rinse brings out the highlights and helps prevent dandruff.

In addition to soothing the nervous system, chamomile's anti-inflammatory properties make it a good remedy for skin problems. An infusion of chamomile can be gently dabbed on the skin to relieve acne and eczema. After washing your face, gently dab it on the affected areas with a cotton ball. In addition, the infusion can be used to clean cuts and scrapes. As an alternative, use the infusion to make a cream for skin problems or for first aid.

New mothers can find relief for sore nipples and mastitis with a warm chamomile poultice gently applied to the area. A hot poultice can ease toothache pain and reduce swelling. It is also effective for earaches. When using a hot poultice, make sure that it is comfortable and not so hot that it burns.

A chamomile infusion or salve is effective for treating itchy rashes and insect bites and stings. Combining lavender and chamomile adds power to your salve and creates a wonderful blend of scents. Use it as first aid for burns, too.

CHAMOMILE AND LAVENDER HEALING INFUSION
2 tablespoons dried chamomile flowers, crumbled
2 tablespoons dried lavender flowers, crumbled
1 cup avocado or olive oil

Combine the herbs and oil in a double boiler. On very low heat, simmer for 30 to 60 minutes. Remove from heat and let cool. Use a stainless steel strainer lined with cheesecloth over a bowl to strain. Fold the cheesecloth over the herbs to press out as much oil as possible.

The calming effects of chamomile are not just for adults. A sleepy-time sachet slipped under a child's pillow or hung from the headboard is a calming aid. The fragrance of the dried flowers can be boosted with a drop or two of essential oil. Also, pop the sachet into the microwave just long enough for the warmth to release more fragrance from the flowers. For toddlers in pain, the Teething Trouble Tonic can help soothe this major sleep disruptor.

CHAMOMILE TEETHING TROUBLE TONIC

6 drops chamomile infusion

2 teaspoons vegetable oil

Combine and mix well. Store in the fridge and when needed take 1 teaspoon of mixture and dilute it with 1 teaspoon of cold water. Mix and then apply a little bit with your finger or a cotton ball to the baby's gums.

....

How to Use the Essential Oils

German chamomile essential oil is inky-blue with a warm, herbaceous, sweet scent. Roman chamomile is pale blue and turns yellow with age. It has a herbaceous, sweet, applelike scent.

Famous as a calming herb, chamomile can help settle a child at bedtime, especially after a busy day. A diffuser with either chamomile essential oil can be used in place of a sachet or sleep pillow.

Instead of using an herbal infusion for skin problems as mentioned above, use chamomile essential oil or blend it with other oils. The diluted essential oil can be dabbed onto problem areas, or use it to make a skin cream.

CHAMOMILE FOR THE SKIN OIL

3 drops chamomile essential oil

2 drops clary essential oil

1 drop rosemary essential oil

1 tablespoon sweet almond carrier oil

Mix the essential oils together and then combine with the carrier oil.

....

The combination of chamomile with clary and rosemary also works well for a massage oil to relieve stress and soothe sore muscles. Roman chamomile is especially good for massage to ease muscle aches and pains, arthritis, rheumatism, and rheumatoid arthritis. Refer to the profile on yarrow for a blend to ease the pain.

Clary: See the Sages

Coriander/Cilantro

(Coriandrum sativum L.)

Also known as: Chinese Parsley, Coriander Seed, Fresh Coriander, Italian Parsley

With their use dating to the Sumerian and Babylonian civilizations, coriander seeds are one of the oldest flavorings in the world. Both the seeds and leaves were used in Egypt and around the Mediterranean region as early as 1500 BCE.[26] The seeds were important enough in Egypt to be included in tombs as food set aside for the afterlife. This plant was listed in the Ebers papyrus and noted in the writings of Hippocrates. The Greeks and Romans used the seeds for medicinal and culinary purposes and enjoyed its taste to flavor wine. Pliny mentioned this plant for a range of ailments. The Romans introduced it into western Europe and Britain.

In Elizabethan England, sugar-coated seeds were served as an after-dinner sweet that did double duty helping digestion and preventing gas. The seeds were used in remedies, mixed with spices for curries, and used to flavor liqueurs. Coriander is an ingredient, along with lemon balm and angelica, in Carmelite water, a digestive aid and tonic first made in the seventeenth century by Carmelite nuns.[27]

Medicinal Uses

Anorexia, anxiety, appetite stimulant, arthritis, bad breath, bloating, cardiovascular system support, digestive system support, fever, flatulence, gastritis, gout, headache, heartburn, indigestion, infection, joint stiffness, lymph circulation, muscle aches and pain, nausea, nerve pain, nervous system support, rheumatism, skin care, stomachache or pain, stomach ulcer, stress, temporomandibular joint pain (TMJ), upset stomach

Precautions and Contraindications

The essential oils: Avoid during pregnancy; use in moderation.

Parts of Plant Used

Herbal remedies: Leaves and seeds

Essential oils: Seeds

Culinary purposes: Leaves, seeds, and roots

---

26. Chevallier, *The Encyclopedia of Medicinal Plants*, 193.
27. Gladstar, *Medicinal Herbs*, 159.

Growing and Harvesting

Coriander/cilantro is a strongly aromatic herb that grows eighteen to twenty-four inches tall on slender, erect stems. The pinnate lower leaves (the familiar cilantro) are rounded and lobed. The upper leaves are feathery and delicate. Tiny white to pale lilac or mauve flowers grow in umbel clusters and bloom from midsummer to early autumn. The ball-shaped, golden-brown seeds are less than ¼ inch in diameter. They grow in clusters and have a musty odor, which changes to warm and spicy as they ripen. The root looks like a long, thin carrot.

Type	Zone	Light	Soil	Moisture	Height	Spacing
Annual	Any	Full sun to partial shade	Any	Dry	18–14"	8–10"

Coriander is an easy-going plant. While it prefers full sun to partial shade, it will do okay in a more shady spot. It is slow to germinate but if you do start it from seed, sow it directly in place as it does not do well when transplanted. Propagate by sowing fresh seeds or let it help you as it readily reseeds, which is why it is sometimes mistaken for a perennial. Coriander is a good companion to anise, caraway, and spinach. It is bad for fennel. This herb repels aphids, beetles, and spider mites. It attracts bees and other pollinators.

You will need several plants if you want to harvest both leaves and seeds. The lower leaves and stems can be harvested when the plant is five to six inches tall or before the flowers bloom. Seeds are generally ready to harvest when the leaves and flowers turn brown. Dried leaves and seeds should be stored separately. The leaves can also be frozen.

How to Use the Herb

The two names of this herb are for different parts of the plant. Coriander refers to the seeds, and cilantro to the lower leaves. In food, both the seeds and leaves enhance the absorption of nutrients and help prevent bloating and flatulence. Coriander seeds have antibacterial and anti-inflammatory properties that fight infection in the digestive tract and help soothe gastritis and stomach ulcers. Also, coriander stimulates the appetite and can aid in dealing with anorexia.

A tea made with either the seeds or leaves eases indigestion, nausea, stomachaches and upsets, and heartburn. Coriander can be combined with fennel seeds for a digestive tea, too. After dinner, chew a few seeds to sweeten the breath, especially after eating garlic, or make a tea with the leaves. Drink coriander tea or use it as a mouthwash to sweeten the breath.

SWEETEN THE BREATH CORIANDER TEA

2–3 tablespoons fresh leaves, chopped

1 cup water

Place the leaves and water in a pan and bring to a boil. Reduce the heat and simmer for 2 to 3 minutes. Steep for 10 minutes and strain.

....

Coriander improves blood circulation, which helps cleanse the body and relieve gout. It also promotes the circulation of lymph. A tea made with the seeds can help break a fever, and a warm poultice of seeds relieves the pain of rheumatism and joint stiffness. Because the leaves have antibacterial and astringent properties, an infusion makes a good facial wash for oily skin to clear blackheads.

This herb is rich in vitamins and minerals and offers good support for the digestive and nervous systems. While only the seeds and leaves are used in remedies, the entire plant is edible. The seeds are like a background spice with an earthy, lemony taste that supports other flavors. The fresh leaves are almost citrus-like, and the roots taste similar to the leaves but with a little nutty flavor. The roots can be chopped and used in stir-fries.

Cilantro, the leaves, may be best known as a common ingredient in salsa, however, they can be used in pesto instead of basil. They can be chopped and sprinkled on cooked foods or added to soups, however, their taste fades with heat so it is best to add them just before serving. Cilantro has a cooling effect, which is why it is so often used in spicy foods. The leaves can be sprinkled into green salads, but sparingly as the flavor can be overwhelming. Cilantro goes well with oregano, ginger, garlic, and cumin.

Coriander seeds are an ingredient in curry powder and they go especially well with cumin. (See the recipe for Spicy Veggie Sprinkle in the profile on cayenne.) Coriander honey makes a nice, warming addition to almost any tea and it can be used as a glaze when roasting meats and vegetables. The taste of the seeds also goes well with vegetables or grain dishes, or combine coriander with other seeds for a spiced butter.

CORIANDER SPICED BUTTER

1 teaspoon fennel seeds

½ teaspoon coriander seeds

½ teaspoon cumin seeds

1 cup butter, margarine, or ghee

Crush or make a powder of the seeds and mix well. Use a fork to cream the butter so it is soft. Add the herbs, and then mix until they are dispersed throughout. Spoon into a container and refrigerate.

....

How to Use the Essential Oils

Coriander essential oil ranges from colorless to pale yellow. Its scent is sweet, spicy, and slightly woody.

Instead of using a poultice to relieve stiff joints, coriander essential oil is an analgesic that eases muscle aches and pains, arthritis, and nerve pain. Combining coriander with rosemary and lemongrass creates an effective oil that also reduces stress. Coriander and rosemary make a good combination for TMJ but be sure to mix a 1 percent dilution for use on the face.

CORIANDER PAIN AWAY MASSAGE OIL

5 drops lemongrass essential oil

4 drops rosemary essential oil

3 drops coriander essential oil

1 ounce carrier oil

Mix the essential oils together and then combine with the carrier oil.

....

Coriander oil is effective for relaxing away stress and anxiety, and relieving headaches. One of the best ways to deal with these issues is a good soak in the tub. Combine coriander with lavender and chamomile to make bath salts that you will probably want to use frequently and not just as a remedy.

CORIANDER SOOTHING SOAK BATH SALTS

5 drops lavender essential oil

4 drops coriander essential oil

4 drops chamomile essential oil

2 cups Epsom or sea salts

Mix the essential oils together. Place the salts in a glass bowl, add the essential oils, and mix thoroughly. Store in a jar with a tight lid.

Dill

(Anethum graveolens L.)

Also known as: American Dill, Dill Weed, Dillseed, Dilly, European Dill, Garden Dill

This herb's common name comes from the Norse *dylla*, meaning to "soothe" or "lull," and its species name *graveolens* is Latin meaning "strong scented."[28] The leaves are often referred to as dill weed. Cultivated for thousands of years, dill has been an important culinary and medicinal herb in many cultures. It was mentioned as a medicinal herb in the ancient Ebers papyrus and other Egyptian writing. Greek physician Dioscorides used it so much for his patients that it became known as "the herb of Dioscorides."[29] Roman writers Pliny and Virgil also mentioned it.

Dill remained a commonly used medicinal and culinary herb through the time of the Renaissance and beyond. European settlers didn't want to leave it behind and brought it with them to North America. In Colonial times, dill seeds were known as "meetin' seeds" because people chewed them during long church meetings to stave off hunger.[30]

Medicinal Uses

Amenorrhea, bad breath, breast problems, breastfeeding problems, bronchitis, chest congestion, colds, colic, cough, digestive system support, flatulence, headache, heartburn, hiccups, indigestion, menstrual cramps, nervous tension, postnatal depression, sleep aid

Precautions and Contraindications

The herb: Avoid in medicinal concentrations during pregnancy (dill pickles are okay).

The essential oils: Avoid during pregnancy.

Parts of Plant Used

Herbal remedies: Leaves and seeds

Essential oils: Leaves and seeds are used for two separate oils

Culinary purposes: Leaves and seeds

---

28. Chevallier, *The Encyclopedia of Medicinal Plants*, 166.
29. Carol Schiller and David Schiller, *The Aromatherapy Encyclopedia: A Concise Guide to Over 385 Plant Oils* (Laguna Beach, CA: Basic Health Publications, 2008), 105.
30. Naomi E. Balaban and James E. Bobick, eds., *The Handy Science Answer Book, 4th ed.* (Canton, MI: Visible Ink Press, 2011), 408.

Growing and Harvesting

Dill looks very similar to its cousin fennel. The way to tell them apart is that dill has one stem whereas fennel has multiple stems. Reaching approximately three feet tall, dill has an erect, hollow stem. The leaves are ferny, thread-like, and blue-green. Large, flat umbel clusters of yellow flowers bloom mid to late summer. The oval seeds are flat and ribbed, and approximately ⅙ inch long. Dill is also related to anise and caraway.

Type	Zone	Light	Soil	Moisture	Height	Spacing
Annual	Any	Full sun	Loam	Average moisture	3'	10–12"

Dill can be grown from seed but it should be started where you want it to grow as it does not transplant well. Propagate it by sowing fresh seeds or let it help you as it readily self-seeds. It grows well in a container.

This herb is good for cabbage, corn, cucumbers, lettuce, and onions. It should not be planted next to carrots or tomatoes. Also avoid planting it near fennel because they will cross-pollinate and produce plants that are neither dill nor fennel and have no medicinal use. Dill repels imported cabbage moths, cabbage loopers, and tomato hornworms. It attracts bees and other beneficial insects. In addition, dill helps deter deer that can ravage a garden.

To use fresh leaves, harvest small bunches after the plant is at least six inches tall. For drying, harvest whole stems just before the plant blooms. Leaves can be hung to dry or cut them from the stems and freeze. For seeds, before the seed heads turn brown enclose them in paper bags and cut the stalks.

How to Use the Herb

In addition to its wonderful taste, dill has been popular in cooking because it soothes the digestive tract. Dill tea, made with 1 or 2 teaspoons of crushed seeds, eases indigestion, heartburn, and flatulence. It also helps to cleanse the liver, and it is good after meals to prevent bad breath. Chewing on a few seeds will also clear the breath.

DILL DIGESTIVE POWER INFUSION

1 tablespoon dried dill leaves, crumbled

1 tablespoon dill seeds, crushed

2 tablespoons dried chamomile flowers, crumbled

2 tablespoons dried peppermint leaves, crumbled

1 quart boiling water

Combine the herbs and add the water. Steep for 30 to 60 minutes and strain.

Drink up to three or four cups a day of the digestive infusion. As an alternative to the infusion, make a tincture with the same combination of herbs and take ½ teaspoon every hour up to 2 teaspoons.

The antispasmodic properties of dill can rescue you from hiccups. However, in a pinch, if you have a jar of dill pickles in the fridge, take half a cup of the liquid and sip a little at a time. Dill water is another treatment to settle the digestive system. Drink half a cup at a time.

DILL WATER

1–2 teaspoons dill seeds

1 pinch salt

1 pint water

Place the seeds in a jar with the salt, add just enough water to cover, and soak for 7 hours. Drain off the water. Boil 1 pint of fresh water, add the seeds, and simmer for 10 minutes. Let it cool and then strain. Stored in the fridge for up to 2 days.

Dill is a warming herb that is helpful during breastfeeding if insufficient milk is a problem. It also aids in easing postnatal depression. Both the seeds and leaves help increase lactation, however, the seeds are more potent and are usually used to make a tea. Use 1 or 2 teaspoons of crushed seeds in 1 cup of boiling water. Drink up to three cups a day. In addition to increasing milk, dill functions as a treatment for breast congestion that sometimes occurs during nursing. The tea taken by nursing mothers will also relieve colic in their babies. In addition, dill seed tea relieves amenorrhea and eases menstrual cramps.

Most famously, dill is known for putting a tang in pickles, but it can be used for so much more because it contains a number of vitamins and minerals that support good health. Dill can liven up almost any dish and make something simple taste sophisticated. It goes well in fish and poultry dishes, breads, cheeses, salads, salad dressing, and a wide range of vegetables.

ALL PURPOSE DILL SAUCE

1 tablespoon fresh dill leaves, finely chopped

or ½ teaspoon dried leaves, crumbled

1½ teaspoons olive oil or lemon juice

1 garlic clove, minced (optional)

Salt and freshly ground pepper, to taste

½ cup plain yogurt

This sauce can be made in a number of ways depending on your taste. Instead of garlic, use a teaspoon of Dijon mustard. Throw in some finely-diced cucumbers, thinly-sliced scallions, or chives chopped into small pieces. Instead of just yogurt as its base, use a half and half mix of yogurt and mayonnaise, or use only sour cream.

....

Dill and garlic go well together for an infused cooking oil. Dill also makes a tangy oil on its own or in a vinegar using a white wine or cider vinegar. Combine dill with borage in a white wine vinegar for a nice complement to salads. For an herb butter, margarine, or ghee combine dill with a pinch of peppermint or spearmint. Also when combining herbs to freeze or store, try dill with parsley and mint, or with lemon balm and mint.

How to Use the Essential Oils

Two oils are produced from the dill plant. The oil from the seeds is colorless to pale yellow with a fresh, warm spicy scent. The oil from the leaves is also colorless to pale yellow but with a sweet spicy scent.

Either essential oil can be used in a diffuser for help in calming nervous tension and for headache relief. Dill also promotes restful sleep. In addition to using a diffuser, try a 2 percent dilution ratio in carrier oil and dab it on your wrists to enjoy the same benefits no matter where you go. As an alternative, combine dill with other essential oils for a healing aromatic treat.

DILL HEADACHE AND TENSION DIFFUSER BLEND

3 drops dill seed or leaf essential oil

2 drops lavender essential oil

1 drop peppermint essential oil

Combine the oils and let the blend mature for about 1 week.

....

Dill seed is the stronger of the two essential oils and is useful for treating colds, bronchitis and other coughs, and chest congestion to get rid of excess mucous. Combine it in equal amounts with peppermint for a soothing steam inhalation.

Fennel

(Foeniculum vulgare, syn. *F. officinale)*

Also known as: Bitter Fennel, Common Fennel, Wild Fennel

The name fennel comes from the ancient Roman word for fragrant hay, *foeniculum.*[31] In the Middle Ages, the name evolved into fanculum and then the plant became known popularly as fenkel.[32]

The Egyptians ate fennel after meals to help with digestion. The Romans and Greeks enjoyed fennel for a range of medicinal and culinary uses. Greek physicians Dioscorides and Hippocrates recommended it for nursing mothers. In China and India, fennel was considered a remedy for snake bites. This herb was widely used during the Middle Ages, and herbalists Culpeper and Gerard recommended it for a range of ailments. In addition to culinary and medicinal purposes, fennel has been used to create brown, green, and yellow dyes.

Medicinal Uses

Amenorrhea, appetite stimulant, belching, bloating, breastfeeding problems, bruises, cellulite, constipation, cough, edema, expectorant, eye problems, flatulence, gout, heartburn, indigestion, kidney stones, lymph circulation, menopausal discomfort, menstrual cycle problems, nasal congestion, nausea, postnatal depression, premenstrual syndrome (PMS), pyorrhea, skin care, sore throat, stomachache or pain, water retention

Precautions and Contraindications

The herb: Avoid during pregnancy; avoid if you have epilepsy or other seizure disorder; use in moderation; should not be given to children under age six.

The essential oils: The herbal precautions also apply; may cause skin irritation in some.

Parts of Plant Used

Herbal remedies: Seeds and leaves

Essential oils: Seeds of a variety called sweet fennel (*Foeniculum vulgare* var. *dulce*)

Culinary purposes: Leaves, bulbs, and seeds

Growing and Harvesting

Reaching four to five feet in height, fennel has a white to creamy colored bulbous base with multiple stalks. The green leaves are feathery and threadlike. Tiny bright yellow flowers grow in large umbel

---

31. Wilson, *Aromatherapy,* 71.

32. Margaret Grieve, *A Modern Herbal, Vol. I* (Mineola, NY: Dover Publications, 1971), 293.

clusters that bloom mid to late summer. The flat, oval seeds are light brown and ridged. They are one quarter to one half inch long. Fennel is a cousin to anise, caraway, and dill.

Type	Zone	Light	Soil	Moisture	Height	Spacing
Perennial	4	Full sun	Sandy or loam	Moderately dry	4–5'	12"

Fennel is a perennial that is often grown as an annual. It prefers full sun but tolerates partial shade in southern areas. South of zone 5 you can sow seeds in the autumn. Propagate this herb by sowing fresh seeds or let it help you as it readily reseeds. Fennel would not win a popularity contest with other plants. It needs to be kept away from bush beans, caraway, tomatoes, and kohlrabi as it will have a negative effect on them. It should not be near dill, either, because they will cross-pollinate and produce plants that are neither dill nor fennel and have no medicinal use. Coriander is harmful to fennel because it prevents seeds from forming. The redeeming factor for fennel is that it repels aphids, slugs, and snails. It attracts lady bugs.

All parts of the plant are edible and can be frozen. Leaves can be harvested any time and hung or screen dried. Watch for seeds to turn from yellow-green to brown. They fall easily so it is usually best to snip off the entire seed head when it begins to turn color and hang it to dry in a bag. The roots can be harvested in the autumn or early spring.

How to Use the Herb

Fennel is a warming herb that is helpful during breastfeeding when insufficient milk is a problem. It also helps ease postnatal depression. Drink up to three cups of tea a day.

> FENNEL MOTHER'S MILK TEA
> 1–2 teaspoons seeds, crushed
> 1 cup boiling water
>
> Pour the water over the seeds and steep for 10 to 15 minutes. Strain and add a little honey to sweeten.

Fennel contains a substance similar to estrogen that helps regulate scanty or painful menstrual cycles. It increases menstrual flow and is an aid for amenorrhea. This herb helps to reduce PMS symptoms, fluid retention, and menopausal discomforts. Overall, it has a toning effect on women's reproductive systems. Also calming, fennel seeds can be combined with chamomile flowers and coriander seeds in equal parts of ½ teaspoon each for a relaxing tea.

The same mild diuretic properties that help reduce premenstrual water retention make fennel helpful in treating gout and kidney stones. In general, it aids in flushing toxins from the body, which is especially helpful for issues with the joints.

Fennel can be used for a wide range of digestive problems including stomachache, constipation, nausea, belching, bloating, flatulence, heartburn, and indigestion. It also stimulates the appetite. Drinking fennel tea is a nice, easy, and comforting way to deal with these digestive issues.

Fennel Digestive Rescue Tea

1–1½ teaspoons seeds, crushed

1 cup boiling water

Pour the water over the seeds and steep for 15 to 20 minutes. Strain before drinking.

....

As an alternative, the tea can be prepared with ½ teaspoon each of fennel seeds, dried peppermint leaves, and/or dried lemon balm leaves. For bloating and flatulence, make a tea with ½ teaspoon of fennel seeds in 1 cup of boiling water and drink up to four cups a day. In addition to tummy troubles, the Digestive Rescue Tea helps ease chronic coughs. It can be used as a gargle for sore throats or as a mouthwash for gum problems such as pyorrhea.

Nowadays we spend a great deal of time staring at computers, smart phones, and a wide range of electronic screens. Whether you just need a break or if your eyes are tired or inflamed, fennel can soothe them. Boil a handful of leaves in 2 cups of water for fifteen minutes. Let it cool to lukewarm, strain, and soak a washcloth for a compress. Place it over your eyes and rest for at least ten minutes.

Like most herbs, fennel is useful for both healing and keeping healthy. With a mild, aniselike flavor, fennel is easy to work into a range of dishes. Fresh or dried leaves can be used in fish dishes, salads, and dressings. When adding the fresh leaves to cooked dishes, do so at the last moment as too much heat tends to destroy their flavor. The next time you make a pasta sauce, try a mixture of dried rosemary, thyme, and fennel.

Pasta Seasoning Mix with Fennel

1 tablespoon dried rosemary, crumbled

1 tablespoon dried thyme, crumbled

1 teaspoon fennel seeds, crushed

Combine ingredients and mix well. Add a little to your pasta sauce and taste as you go to get a flavor balance that you like.

....

While the fennel bulb is also used in a range of dishes such as seafood, chicken, and roasted root vegetables, it is quite yummy on its own. Slice it vertically in half and drizzle with a little olive oil. Sprinkle with grated Parmesan cheese and bread crumbs, and then bake for about thirty minutes at 400° Fahrenheit. This makes a nice complement to tomato-based pasta dishes.

How to Use the Essential Oils

The seeds of sweet fennel produce a yellow to pale orange-brown oil. It has an herby, spicy, anise-like scent.

Using this essential oil for massage helps to increase lymph circulation, decrease cellulite, and reduce the swelling associated with edema. Fennel essential oil also helps tone the skin. Use 7 or 8 drops in 1 ounce of carrier oil, or try a soothing blend with lavender and rosemary.

FENNEL MASSAGE OIL BLEND

6 drops fennel essential oil

4 drops lavender essential oil

3 drops rosemary essential oil

1 ounce carrier oil

Mix the essential oils together and then combine with the carrier oil.

Fennel on its own in a carrier oil can be used to treat bruises. In addition, its antibacterial and anti-inflammatory properties make it effective to use as a steam inhalation to relieve nasal congestion and reduce excess mucous. This will also help soothe coughs.

Garlic

(Allium sativum L.)

Also known as: Common Garlic, Poor Man's Treacle, Stinking Rose, Stinkweed

The use of garlic was recorded approximately five thousand years ago in Sumer (present-day Iraq).[33] Garlic was also used by the Babylonians and throughout the Middle East. It was used in China as early as 2000 BCE.[34] In Egypt, it was an important part of the diet as well as the medicine chest. The Spartans of ancient Greece also included garlic in their daily diet. Mentioned by Pliny, the Romans valued this plant as a food to give their soldiers strength.

Garlic is the main ingredient in Four Thieves Vinegar, a remedy popular in France since the early eighteenth century. The name of this vinegar comes from the story about four criminals whose punishment was to bury plague victims in Marseilles. The fact that the men never got sick was attributed to their eating crushed garlic in wine vinegar. During World War I, garlic was used on the battlefield to clean infected wounds and to treat dysentery.

On a personal note, one of my favorite restaurants in San Francisco is the Stinking Rose where their motto is to "season garlic with food."

Medicinal Uses

Athlete's foot, blood pressure, blood sugar, bronchitis, cardiovascular system support, cholesterol, colds, coughs, digestive system support, ear infection, flu, immune system support, infection, insect bites and stings, jock itch, ringworm, sinusitis, sore throats, staph infection, sties, strep throat, tonsillitis, vaginal yeast infection (vaginitis), warts

Precautions and Contraindications

The herb: May cause heartburn or irritate the stomach in some; avoid when nursing; garlic applied directly to the skin may cause burns.

The essential oils: Use in small amounts and well diluted; may cause sensitization in some.

Part of Plant Used

Herbal remedies, essential oils, and culinary purposes: Cloves

Growing and Harvesting

Reaching one to two feet high, garlic has long, flat, pointed leaves that grow from a single stem sprouting from the bulb. The bulb usually contains four to fifteen separate fleshy sections called

---

33. Bonar, *Herbs*, 68.
34. Kowalchik, *Rodale's Illustrated Encyclopedia of Herbs*, 215.

cloves, which are enclosed in white, papery skin. A cluster of fibrous roots is attached to the bottom of the bulb. Separate leafless stems produce clusters of small white to pinkish flowers in a globe-shaped umbel. The flowers bloom from late spring to early summer.

Type	Zone	Light	Soil	Moisture	Height	Spacing
Perennial	4	Full sun	Loam	Moderately moist	1–2'	6'

Garlic is a perennial that lasts several years, however, it is grown as an annual for harvesting. It grows best in well-composted soil, and it is easier to start from individual cloves than from seeds. Plant the cloves, pointed end up, approximately two inches deep in the autumn or early spring. A new bulb will form around each clove. Garlic does well when grown in a container. To produce bigger bulbs, cut back the flowering stalks. Garlic is propagated by sowing new cloves or seeds.

Garlic attracts butterflies and repels slugs, snails, Japanese beetles, aphids, and ants. It can also deter rabbits. In the vegetable garden garlic is a good companion to peas, cabbage, celery, cucumbers, eggplants, lettuce, and tomatoes. It is especially beneficial near fruit trees and roses.

Harvest the bulbs by digging them out when the lower leaves begin to turn brown and fall over. The whole bulb can be hung to dry with roots and stem attached. The leaves of multiple plants are often braided together to make a rope of garlic bulbs.

Drying will take three to four weeks. When the outer skin becomes papery, they're dry. The roots can be cut off and the stem cut an inch or two from the bulb. Store them in a mesh bag in a cool, dark place and they will last for several months. For long-term storage, peel the cloves and cut them into slices. These can be dried like roots, and then stored or made into a powder. After the harvest, save some cloves at room temperature to plant your next crop.

How to Use the Herb

The antiviral and antibacterial properties of garlic make it an excellent choice for treating colds, flu, and sinusitis. The compounds that are excreted through the lungs and cause garlic breath actually put the healing components right where they are needed for respiratory illnesses. Cooked garlic is effective but raw cloves are more potent. (You may want to keep anise, fennel, or dill seeds, or parsley leaves on hand for your breath.) A syrup may make the garlic more palatable while it soothes a sore or strep throat, tonsillitis, cough, and bronchitis. Take a teaspoon of syrup at a time throughout the day. Garlic is also effective for fighting staph infections.

GARLIC SYRUP

2–3 cloves, crushed

4 tablespoons honey

Wrap the garlic in a piece of muslin or cheesecloth, crush it, and place in a jar. Cover the garlic with honey and let it stand for 2 to 3 hours. Stir and remove the garlic.

....

Garlic in the diet helps to boost the immune system so eating it throughout the cold and flu season is beneficial. Or, if you have powdered garlic and prefer capsules, take one twice a day.

The blood-thinning effect of eating garlic supports the cardiovascular system and helps reduce the risk of heart attack. It helps to slightly lower high blood pressure, too. Used regularly in cooking, garlic reduces and helps maintain healthy cholesterol levels and lowers blood sugar levels. Garlic is an aid to poor or sluggish digestion, too. Eating garlic is also a treatment for sties and it can help cure an infection of the middle ear.

Pesto is a tasty way to include garlic in the diet. So is olive oil infused with rosemary, thyme, and garlic, which is great for cooking. And, of course, garlic butter to top warm bread served with pasta dishes. However, roasted garlic is the ultimate comfort food, in my opinion. It can be used in so many dishes, or just slice the cloves and eat them on a thick piece of crusty French or Italian bread... *magnifique!*

Roasted Garlic
Several garlic bulbs
Olive oil

Leave the bulbs intact for roasting. Hold a bulb on its side and slice off enough of the top so each clove is cut open. Lightly coat a shallow baking dish or muffin tin with olive oil and arrange the bulbs inside. Drizzle with oil and then spread it around, coating the top of each clove. Sprinkle with a little sea salt and pepper, cover with aluminum foil, and bake at 375° Fahrenheit for 35 to 45 minutes. Allow to cool enough to handle, and then squeeze each bulb from the bottom to push out the cloves or use a small fork to extract them.

....

Garlic's infection-fighting powers extend to fungal and yeast infections. For athlete's foot, crush a clove, place it in a jar, and pour in a cup of olive oil. Let it sit for two days and then strain. Use a cotton swab to apply the oil to the affected areas. This oil can also be used to treat ringworm, warts, jock itch, and insect bites and stings. Never apply garlic directly to the skin as it can cause burns.

Garlic Vaginitis Treatment
1 teaspoon garlic juice
2 tablespoons yogurt

Use a garlic press to squeeze the juice out of several cloves and mix well with yogurt. To use the vaginitis treatment, soak a tampon in the mixture for 10 minutes. Insert it before bed and remove it in the morning. The yogurt acts as a soothing medium for the garlic juice to avoid burns. Do this each night while symptoms last. This remedy may be smelly but it is effective. It is important to catch a yeast infection in its early stages for home treatment. See your doctor if the condition persists.

....

How to Use the Essential Oils

Garlic essential oil can range from colorless to pale yellow. And, as you might expect, it smells like garlic.

If you don't want to eat garlic but would like its benefits when you have a cold or other respiratory ailment, the essential oil can help in a steam inhalation. Start with 2 drops of essential oil in a quart of boiling water. If it is not overwhelming, go to 3 drops. Inhaling the steam will put the garlic where it is needed—in your lungs. It will also detoxify the body and disinfect the air in the room.

The essential oil can be used instead of the infused oil for topical treatments, however, it must be well diluted. Do not use more than 1 drop in 3 ounces of carrier oil.

Hyssop

(Hyssopus officinalis L.)

Also known as: Hedge Hyssop

Hyssop was highly regarded as a medicinal herb by the ancient Greeks and Romans who also used it for domestic cleaning. In addition, the Romans used the leaves for culinary purposes, including a wine they called *Hyssopites*.[35] The plant and the wine were mentioned by Pliny. Hippocrates recommended hyssop for chest problems, and Dioscorides recommended it to treat a number of conditions.

By the tenth century, hyssop had been introduced throughout Europe by Benedictine monks who used it for making liqueurs. It is an ingredient in Benedictine, an herbal liqueur that was developed as an elixir by a Benedictine monk in 1510.[36] The secret recipe was lost but then rediscovered in the nineteenth century.

During the Middle Ages, hyssop was commonly used as a strewing herb as well as stuffing material for mattresses. Small branches of hyssop were used by Roman Catholic priests to dip in holy water and sprinkle blessings on their congregations. The common name "hedge hyssop" comes from its use as a clipped hedging plant in knot gardens.

Medicinal Uses

Anxiety, asthma, bloating, bronchitis, bruises, catarrh, chest congestion, cold sores, colds, cough, cuts and scrapes, dermatitis, digestive system support, eczema, expectorant, fever, flatulence, flu, herpes, indigestion, infection, inflammation, insect repellent, nasal congestion, nervous system support, nervous tension, skin care, sore throat, stress, tonsillitis

Precautions and Contraindications

The herb: Avoid during pregnancy and while nursing; avoid in children under eighteen; use in small doses for short periods of time.

The essential oils: Herbal precautions also apply; should not be used by epileptics or those with any type of seizure disorder; avoid with high blood pressure; may cause sensitization in some.

Parts of Plant Used

Herbal remedies: Leaves, stems, and flowers

Essential oils: Leaves and flower buds

Culinary purposes: Leaves

---

35. Denys J. Charles, *Antioxidant Properties of Spices, Herbs and Other Sources* (New York: Springer Science and Business Media, 2013), 353.

36. Judyth A. McLeod, *In a Unicorn's Garden: Recreating the Mystery and Magic of Medieval Gardens* (London: Murdoch Books UK Limited, 2008), 252.

Growing and Harvesting

Hyssop has upright, angular stems and reaches about two feet in height. Like other members of the mint family, the stems have a square shape. The leaves are dark green and lance-shaped. Tiny purple-blue flowers grow in whorls at the ends of the stems. They bloom from midsummer to early autumn.

Type	Zone	Light	Soil	Moisture	Height	Spacing
Perennial	4	Full sun to partial shade	Sandy or loam	Moderately dry	2'	12"

It is usually easiest to purchase a plant because the seeds are slow to germinate. Hyssop prefers full sun but will tolerate partial shade. The stems, flowers, and leaves are strongly aromatic, and the leaves have a mintlike smell when crushed. Propagate this herb by root division, stem cuttings, or sowing fresh seeds if you have the patience.

Hyssop is known as a good bee plant. Beekeepers often grow it near their hives because hyssop flower nectar enhances the taste of honey. In addition to bees, it attracts butterflies and humming-birds, and it repels fleas, beetles, cabbage loopers, and imported cabbage moths. Hyssop is a good companion to cabbage and grapes.

Harvest the leaves before flowers appear. If you are harvesting flowers, take them when they are half open. Leaves and flowers can be hung to dry.

How to Use the Herb

Hyssop is a powerful herb with antiviral and antibacterial properties, making it effective for a range of respiratory problems such as colds, bronchitis, and the flu. As an expectorant, it helps clear and cleanse the lungs and fight infection. It also relieves bronchial spasms. Combine hyssop with peppermint for the added benefit of menthol.

HYSSOP AND PEPPERMINT CLEANSING TEA

1½ teaspoons dried hyssop leaves and flowers, crumbled

½ teaspoon dried peppermint leaves, crumbled

1 cup boiling water

Combine the herbs and add the water. Steep 10 to 15 minutes and strain. Add honey to taste.

In addition to the combination of hyssop and peppermint to make a tea, these herbs work well for a steam inhalation to help clear the nasal passages. They also make a good chest rub ointment. Hyssop on its own as a facial steam cleanses the skin.

Plain hyssop tea helps ease asthma attacks, however, the leaves have a minty but slightly bitter flavor, so you may want to add a little honey. The tea can also be used as a gargle to soothe sore throats including tonsillitis. Instead of honey, add a little lemon juice, which will also help your throat. A variation of the tea for bronchitis uses equal amounts of anise seeds, hyssop, and thyme. To encourage sweating and break a fever, make a hyssop infusion and drink half a cup every two hours over a six-hour period. For colds and flu, drink a little at a time up to two cups a day.

When dealing with chronic catarrh, make an infusion with the leaves, stems, and flowers. Flavor it with honey or lemon, and drink one to three cups a day. When you have a cold or the flu, make an infusion of hyssop, peppermint, rosemary, and thyme for a warming, cleansing bath. The steamy vapors will help clear congestion.

CONGESTION-CLEARING HYSSOP BATH INFUSION

1 cup dried hyssop leaves and/or flowers, crumbled

½ cup dried peppermint leaves, crumbled

¼ cup dried rosemary leaves, crumbled

¼ cup dried thyme leaves, crumbled

2 quarts boiling water

Combine the herbs and then add the water. Steep for 1 to 2 hours, strain, and add to bath water.

....

For coughs, infuse hyssop leaves, stems, and flowers or just the flowers to make a syrup. Take a teaspoon of the syrup as needed. Hyssop helps to thin thick mucus and get rid of it. Also, hyssop combines well with thyme to make a cough syrup.

A poultice of fresh chopped leaves helps to heal cuts and bruises. Hyssop can be combined with crushed caraway seeds for this purpose, too. In addition, a hyssop poultice or compress reduces the swelling and bruising of a black eye.

Like many herbs in the mint family, hyssop aids digestion, especially digesting fats. Combine it with two of its cousins, lemon balm and spearmint, for a healthy after-dinner tea.

HYSSOP DIGESTIVE TEA

1 teaspoon dried hyssop leaves and/or flowers, crumbled

½ teaspoon dried spearmint leaves, crumbled

½ teaspoon dried lemon balm leaves, crumbled

1 cup boiling water

Combine the herbs and add the water. Steep for 10 to 15 minutes and strain.

....

A tincture of hyssop is another way to deal with indigestion as well as gas and bloating especially due to nervous tension. Take one half to one teaspoon two or three times a day. The tincture also serves as a tonic to support the nervous system.

For culinary purposes, use fresh hyssop leaves to season poultry dishes, soups, and casseroles. A little of this herb goes a long way as its minty flavor can be somewhat strong, and too much can produce a bitter taste. Experiment using small amounts.

For the home, hyssop is useful as a pest repellent. In the linen closet, use fresh or dried leaves in a sachet to repel moths. Hyssop can also be used in your pet's bedding area to discourage fleas. Make sure it is placed safely out of your pet's reach.

How to Use the Essential Oils

The color of hyssop essential oil ranges from clear to pale yellow to reddish-amber. It has a rich, spicy sweet scent.

In addition to using a tincture as a tonic for the nervous system, hyssop essential oil is an aid for relaxation to quell anxiety, nervous tension, and stress. Use it in a diffuser along with lavender and lemon balm to soothe away tension. Also use this combination in a diffuser or vaporizer during cold and flu season to cleanse the air and treat congestion. In addition, refer to the profile on thyme for an inhaler blend with hyssop.

HYSSOP CLEANSING RELAXATION DIFFUSER BLEND

4 drops hyssop essential oil

4 drops lemon balm essential oil

2 drops lavender essential oil

Combine the oils and let the blend mature for about 1 week.

....

The antiseptic and antiviral properties of hyssop are useful in treating herpes and can inhibit the growth of sores. It also works on common cold sores. Mix 1 drop of essential oil in 1 teaspoon of carrier oil and apply with a cotton swab. It can also be used to relieve the inflammation of dermatitis and other forms of eczema.

Lavender

(Lavandula angustifolia, syn. *L. officinalis)*

Also known as: Common Lavender, English Lavender, Garden Lavender, True Lavender

Lavender has been a well-known and loved fragrance since ancient times. It has been used as an ingredient in cosmetics and perfumery as well as many domestic applications. The Greeks and Romans used it for treating a range of ailments and for cleaning their homes. As mentioned in the introduction to this book, the name lavender comes from the Latin *lavare,* meaning "to wash." The Romans introduced the plant into England where it has become a mainstay in gardens.

Throughout Europe during the Middles Ages, lavender was popular for medicinal purposes as well as a strewing herb to freshen homes, especially sickrooms. Sachets of lavender were used to scent linens and to deter moths, fleas, and other pests. Soap maker William of Yardley knew a good thing when he saw it (or smelled it) and managed to get a monopoly on England's lavender during the 1770s.

This beloved garden plant was imported to North America by the Pilgrims. When French chemist René-Maurice Gattefossé rediscovered its powerful healing properties, lavender came full circle as an important medicinal herb.

Medicinal Uses

Acne, anxiety, athlete's foot, bloating, boils, bronchitis, bruises, burns, chest congestion, chronic fatigue, cold sores, colds, cuts and scrapes, dermatitis, eczema, flatulence, flu, head lice, headache, hemorrhoids, herpes, indigestion, inflammation, insect bites and stings, insomnia, jock itch, joint stiffness, laryngitis, menstrual cramps, migraine, muscle aches and pain, muscle strain, nail fungus, nerve pain, nervous tension, psoriasis, rheumatism, ringworm, scabies, scars, sciatica, sinusitis, skin care, sleep aid, sore throat, sprains, strep throat, stress, sunburn, tonsillitis, vaginal yeast infection (vaginitis)

Precautions and Contraindications

The herb and essential oils: Do not use when taking sedative medications.

Parts of Plant Used

Herbal remedies: Leaves and flowers

Essential oils: Leaves, flowers, and buds

Culinary purposes: Leaves and flowers

Growing and Harvesting

Lavender is a bushy, evergreen shrub that reaches two or three feet in height and spreads about two feet wide. The lower stems of mature plants are usually dense and woody. Small purplish-lavender colored flowers grow in whorls atop leafless spikes. They bloom from midsummer to early autumn. The slightly fuzzy leaves are narrow and gray-green or silvery green.

Type	Zone	Light	Soil	Moisture	Height	Spacing
Perennial	5	Full sun to partial shade	Slightly sandy loam	Dry	2–3'	12–24"

Lavender has been a garden favorite for centuries, which is understandable because it is highly aromatic and makes working or sitting nearby a delightful pleasure. It prefers full sun but tolerates partial shade, and grows well in containers. Propagate this plant by stem cuttings or root division. Lavender is a good companion to daylilies, dianthus, coreopsis, yarrow, and yucca. It's no surprise that lavender attracts bees and butterflies.

Harvest flower spikes and stems when the flowers are almost open. Cut the stem several inches below the flowers and hang them to air dry. They can also be dried on screens. The dried flowers and leaves will remain aromatic for a long time.

How to Use the Herb

There are several types of lavender, which makes it important to purchase the right one for the purposes described here. For example, Spanish or French lavender (*Lavandula stoechas*) is stimulating and has the opposite effect of *Lavandula angustifolia*, the lavender covered in this book.

As an herb, lavender is most widely known for its calming and soothing properties. For a sleep aid and help dealing with insomnia, make a tincture and take one half to one teaspoon with water an hour before bed to improve sleep quality. A little sleep pillow stuffed with lavender flowers also helps to calm and relax. Put the pillow in the microwave just long enough to warm the flowers to release more of their scent.

Lavender tincture or tea has a calming effect, which helps to quell nervous tension. The tincture is also effective in treating migraines and reducing the symptoms of chronic fatigue. A tea made with equal amounts of lavender and lemon balm relieves other types of headaches, especially those caused by tension. In addition, the tea can be used for a warm compress to place on the back of the neck, or let it cool and apply a compress across the forehead and temples, which will also help relieve a headache.

Lavender honey is wonderful in a cup of chamomile tea for a relaxing treat. Make the honey with lavender and lemon balm for added flavor, aroma, and healing. A little spearmint can be added, as well.

LAVENDER AND LEMON BALM HONEY

½ cup fresh lavender flowers, chopped

¼ cup fresh lemon balm leaves, chopped

a pinch of fresh spearmint leaves, chopped

1 cup honey

Pour the honey into a slightly larger mason jar and set in a saucepan of water. Warm over low heat until the honey becomes a little less viscous. Add the herbs and stir with a butter knife to distribute. Continue warming for 15 to 20 minutes, then remove from heat. Put the lid on when cool. Store out of the light at room temperature for a week. Reheat slightly to strain out herbs.

....

Lavender's calming properties extend to the digestive system. Drink half a cup of lavender tea twice a day to soothe indigestion, flatulence, and bloating. Lavender tincture or tea also eases menstrual cramps.

The popularity of lavender soap is not only because of its scent, but because this herb is especially healing for the skin. An infusion for the bath can soothe irritated skin and many other problems as well as relieve muscle and nerve pain. The combination of herbs in the Healing Lavender Bath Infusion also makes an excellent foot soak. In addition, this combination of herbs can be used to make a medicinal honey that is especially soothing in a bedtime cup of tea.

HEALING LAVENDER BATH INFUSION

1 cup dried lavender leaves and flowers, crumbled

½ cup dried chamomile flowers, crumbled

½ cup dried lemon balm leaves, crumbled

2 quarts boiling water

Combine the herbs and then add the water. Steep for 1 to 2 hours. Strain and add to bath water.

....

Lavender has powerful antiseptic and antibacterial properties that make it ideal for a facial steam. In addition to a steam, use an infusion of lavender as a facial rinse to cleanse and stimulate circulation to the skin, heal blemishes, and soothe the inflammation of acne. The infusion is also generally good for oily skin. For additional help in getting rid of acne blemishes, make a vinegar with lavender flowers and leaves, and dab it on the pustules. For sunburn, use an oil infusion or make a cream to soothe and heal the skin.

While the essential oil is particularly good for topical antiviral applications, a strong infusion of the herb can be used to treat vaginitis. Use the infusion for a sitz bath or to make an ointment. The sitz bath or ointment is also effective to reduce the inflammation and pain of hemorrhoids.

This herb can help you get through the cold and flu season, too. Lavender relieves the congestion of sinusitis, bronchitis, and other respiratory problems. One of the best ways is with a steam inhalation, which not only helps to clear the airways but also helps to cleanse the air in the room. To soothe a sore throat, laryngitis, tonsillitis, or strep throat, make an infusion with equal parts of lavender and peppermint. When it cools, pour it into a spray bottle that has a fine mister and use it as a throat spray. The same infusion can be used to make a warm chest compress or make an oil infusion for a chest rub ointment.

LAVENDER HERB AND SALT GARGLE

1 teaspoon dried lavender flowers, crumbled

1 teaspoon dried sage leaves, crumbled

½ teaspoon table salt

1 cup boiling water

Combine the herbs, pour in the water, and steep for 10 minutes. Strain into a mug with the salt. Heat slightly in microwave and stir to dissolve salt.

....

How to Use the Essential Oils

Lavender essential oil is clear with a slight tinge of yellow. It has a mellow, floral, herbaceous scent and balsamic woody undertones.

As mentioned, French chemist René-Maurice Gattefossé rediscovered the soothing and healing power of lavender essential oil after burning his hand in the laboratory. Make an ointment to keep on hand for burns, cuts, and scrapes. Lavender is a skin rejuvenator that relieves pain and heals without scarring. It is also effective for healing acne, boils, and bruises.

LAVENDER FIRST-AID OINTMENT

¼–½ cup jojoba or beeswax

1 cup carrier oil

2 teaspoons lavender essential oil

Place the jojoba or beeswax in a mason jar in a saucepan of water. Warm over low heat until it begins to melt; add the carrier oil. Stir gently for about 15 minutes. Remove from heat, add the essential oil, and stir. Test the thickness by placing a little on a plate and letting it cool in the fridge for a minute or two. If you want it firmer, add more jojoba or beeswax. If it's too thick, add a tiny bit of oil. Let it cool and then store in a cool, dark place.

....

The concentration of lavender's antiseptic, anti-inflammatory, antiviral, and antibacterial properties in the essential oil makes it perfect for a wide range of topical applications. Although it is considered one of the safest essential oils, it is best to use it diluted with a carrier oil.

Lavender relieves the itching and inflammation of athlete's foot and jock itch. It is instrumental for other viral infections such as cold sores, herpes outbreaks, and nail fungus. Use the ointment to soothe the inflammation of skin disorders such as psoriasis, eczema, and dermatitis, too. Lavender can also be used to treat insect bites and stings, head lice, ringworm, and scabies.

Not only does lavender make a great massage oil for relaxing, its analgesic properties make it especially effective to relieve rheumatic pain, sciatica, joint stiffness, muscle aches and strains, and sprains. Sweet almond makes a good carrier oil for this. In addition to massage, use lavender in the bath by mixing 5 drops of essential oil with 1 cup of sea or Epsom salts. For a warm compress, mix 2 drops of essential oil in 1 quart of hot water.

For a sleep aid, sprinkle a little essential oil onto bed linens to surround yourself with the scent. To relieve anxiety and stress, use lavender oil on its own in a diffuser or blend it with rosemary and chamomile.

DIFFUSE YOUR STRESS LAVENDER BLEND

6 drops lavender essential oil

3 drops rosemary essential oil

2 drops chamomile essential oil

Combine the oils and let the blend mature for about 1 week.

Lemon Balm

(Melissa officinalis L.)

Also known as: Bee Balm, Common Balm, Honey Balm, Melissa, Mint Balm, Sweet Balm

The name *Melissa* is Greek and means "bee." [37] Lemon balm attracts and calms bees, which is why beekeepers have grown it near their hives for more than two thousand years. Lemon balm honey has been highly valued since ancient times and was mentioned by both Pliny and Dioscorides, who said it helped to heal wounds. In the eleventh century, Arab physician Avicenna also sung its praises.

Lemon balm was an important medicinal herb in Europe during the Middle Ages and was one of several plants that became known as a cure-all. Even though English herbalists such as Culpeper and Gerard touted its uses, lemon balm's popularity was not carried to the New World. It had to wait for the resurgence of interest in herbal remedies to be rediscovered. Lemon balm earned its name because of its honey-sweet lemon flavor and fragrance.

Medicinal Uses

Acne, anxiety, asthma, blood pressure, bronchitis, chest congestion, colds, cough, dermatitis, digestive system support, eczema, fever, flu, headache, herpes, immune system support, indigestion, infection, inflammation, insect bites and stings, insomnia, menstrual cramps, migraine, nervous system support, premenstrual syndrome (PMS), psoriasis, restlessness, seasonal affective disorder (SAD), shingles, skin care, sleep aid, stomachache or pain, stress

Precautions and Contraindications

The herb: May interact with sedatives and thyroid medications.

The essential oils: May cause skin irritation or sensitization in some.

Parts of Plant Used

Herbal remedies: Leaves and stems

Essential oils: Leaves, flowers, and buds

Culinary purposes: Leaves

Growing and Harvesting

Reaching one to three feet tall, lemon balm is a bushy herb with square, branching stems. Its bright green leaves are deeply veined and have toothed edges. The leaves have a noticeable lemony scent

---

37. Michael Castleman, *The New Healing Herbs: The Classic Guide to Nature's Best Medicines* (Emmaus, PA: Rodale Press, 2001), 305.

especially when brushed against. Small white to yellowish flowers grow in clusters where leaves join the main stems. They bloom from midsummer to early autumn.

Type	Zone	Light	Soil	Moisture	Height	Spacing
Perennial	4	Full sun to partial shade	Loam or sandy loam	Moderately moist	1–3'	12–24"

Lemon balm does well in partial to filtered shade in southern zones but prefers full sun in northern areas. During the first season, the plant may seem scrawny but it will fill out in its second year. Lemon balm is easy to grow in containers. Lemon balm can be propagated by root division, stem cuttings and layering, and by sowing fresh seeds. While its roots will not take over your garden, it does readily self-seed and can become invasive. Keep an eye on it, especially if you let it reseed. Lemon balm attracts bees and is a good companion to squash and pumpkins because it repels squash bugs.

Both the leaves and stems can be harvested throughout the growing season. It can be cut back to two inches above the ground, which will encourage a second crop. The leaves keep their scent when dried, however, they darken if not dried quickly so you may want to avoid hang drying them. As an alternative, freezing works well.

How to Use the Herb

Anytime you want an herbal tea, lemon balm is enjoyable, but after a hectic day, it can seem magical. It calms both the nervous and digestive systems, quelling anxiety and nervous indigestion. This herb eases headaches, lowers blood pressure, and relieves insomnia. Drink the tea an hour or two before going to bed for help in falling asleep.

SIMPLY LEMON BALM TEA

2 teaspoons dried leaves and stems, crumbled

1 cup boiling water

Pour the water over the herb, steep 10 to 15 minutes, and then strain.

For headaches, let the tea steep until it's cool and then drink one cup three times during the day. When dealing with a migraine, use lemon balm on its own or make the tea with 1½ teaspoons of lemon balm and ½ teaspoon of valerian. This combination of herbs is also effective as a sleep aid. Be sure to read the precautions in the profile on valerian.

The tea is an aid for stomach pains, too. To boost its effectiveness for this purpose, use 2 teaspoons each of dried lemon balm, chamomile, and peppermint in 1 cup of water. Brew a mild tea with just 1 teaspoon of lemon balm to soothe restlessness in children.

When suffering from anxiety, try half a teaspoon of lemon balm tincture in one cup of water three times a day. The tea also relieves PMS symptoms and menstrual cramps. Equally effective for headache and anxiety is a tea made with 1 teaspoon of each of lemon balm and chamomile. Brew an infusion with equal amounts of lemon balm, lavender, and chamomile for the bath to soak away stress. Combine lemon balm with equal amounts of St. John's wort in a tea to relieve seasonal affective disorder (SAD).

The antiviral properties of lemon balm make it useful in treating herpes and shingles. It relieves the pain and discomfort, and shortens the length and intensity of outbreaks. Brew the Simply Lemon Balm Tea and drink two or three cups a day. Also, use a little of the tea on a cotton ball to apply directly to sores. An ointment made with jojoba and an infusion of lemon balm applied several times a day is also helpful.

For acne, make a vinegar of herbs to dab on pustules, which will reduce inflammation, counter infection, and fight bacteria. Also use this combination of herbs (without vinegar) for a facial steam to help with acne or to use as a general skin cleanser.

LEMON BALM HERBAL ACNE VINEGAR

3 teaspoons dried rosemary leaves, crumbled

2 teaspoons dried lemon balm leaves, crumbled

2 teaspoons dried lavender flowers, crumbled

2 teaspoons dried chamomile flowers, crumbled

¼–½ cup vinegar

Place the herbs in a jar and pour in enough vinegar to cover them. Steep for at least 2 weeks and strain.

The antiviral components in lemon balm make it ideal to ease the symptoms of colds and flu. Combine it with equal amounts of peppermint for a tea to calm coughs, ease asthma attacks, and relieve congestion due to bronchitis. Also use these two herbs for a steam inhalation to help clear the airways. On its own, a lemon balm tea promotes sweating to reduce fever.

Because the antioxidants in lemon balm help support and strengthen the immune system, use a medicinal honey throughout the cold and flu season to help you stay healthy.

STAY HEALTHY LEMON BALM HONEY

4 tablespoons dried lemon balm leaves, crumbled

3 tablespoons dried chamomile flowers, crumbled

1 tablespoon dried lavender flowers, crumbled

1 cup honey

Pour the honey into a slightly larger jar and set it in a saucepan of water. Warm over low heat until the honey becomes a little less viscous. Add the herbs and stir with a butter knife to distribute. Continue warming for 15 to 20 minutes, then remove from heat. Put the lid on when cool. Store out of the light at room temperature for a week. Reheat slightly to strain herbs or leave them in.

....

Lemon balm is a delightful culinary herb. Sprinkle a few leaves in salads or use them to flavor fish or poultry dishes. Freeze some chopped leaves in ice cube trays to add to drinks. Also when combining herbs to freeze or store together, combine it with dill or mint.

How to Use the Essential Oils

Lemon balm essential oil ranges from pale yellow to full yellow in color. As expected, its scent is lemony but also fresh and herbaceous.

Just as lemon balm tea can be used for herpes and shingles, so too can the essential oil. Mix 1 drop of essential oil in 1 teaspoon of carrier oil and apply to affected areas. This can also be used to relieve the swelling and itching of insect bites and stings. For extra power, blend lemon balm with lavender and St. John's wort and keep some on hand for first aid.

LEMON BALM SOOTHING SKIN RELIEF OIL

6 drops lemon balm essential oil

5 drops lavender essential oil

2 drops St. John's wort essential oil

1 ounce apricot kernel carrier oil

Mix the essential oils together and then combine with the carrier oil.

....

To calm the inflammation and itching of eczema, psoriasis, or dermatitis mix lemon balm with borage as the carrier oil to soothe the skin. Alternatively, mix the essential oil with sea or Epson salts for a healing soak in the tub. Lemon balm is also effective in a diffuser or with a carrier oil for a calming massage to reduce anxiety, headache, and blood pressure.

Lemongrass

(Cymbopogon citratus)

Also known as: Citronella Grass, Madagascar Lemongrass, West Indian Lemongrass

Lemongrass has been cultivated for centuries as a culinary and medicinal herb. It has a long history of use in India for treating fever and infectious diseases. It was also used to freshen the home. As its species name implies, it has a citruslike scent, which may be familiar to many of us who grew up using Ivory® soap. It is an important flavoring ingredient in many Asian cuisines, especially Thai. Lemongrass is also a component in many Ayurvedic remedies.

Medicinal Uses

Acne, arthritis, athlete's foot, digestive system support, fever, flatulence, gastroenteritis, head lice, headache, indigestion, insect bites and stings, insect repellent, jock itch, laryngitis, mental fatigue, muscle ache or pain, nerve pain, nervous exhaustion, rheumatism, ringworm, scabies, skin care, sore throat, sprains, stomachache or pain, stress, vaginal yeast infection (vaginitis)

Precautions and Contraindications

The essential oils: May cause skin irritation; do not use around the eyes; do not use on babies or children; avoid during pregnancy; may cause dermal irritation or sensitization in some.

Parts of Plant Used

Herbal remedies and essential oils: Leaves

Culinary purposes: Stems

Growing and Harvesting

Lemongrass is a tropical aromatic grass with a pungent, lemony fragrance. It grows in large, dense clumps that can reach up to five feet tall and four feet wide. Lemongrass has long, narrow leaf blades. The base of the leaf stems are white and enlarged, similar to leeks. Inconspicuous, greenish flowers grow atop branching stalks, however, lemongrass rarely comes into bloom.

Type	Zone	Light	Soil	Moisture	Height	Spacing
Perennial	9	Full sun	Sandy loam	Moist	3–5'	2–4'

If you are in the warmer zones, lemongrass can be started by seed. For container growing in cooler zones, start seeds in six-inch pots. To overwinter indoors, give it a warm, sunny location. This plant is most easily propagated by root division. Lemongrass repels ants, flies, and mosquitoes. It is a good companion to lavender, mints, and sage.

The leaves and stems can be harvested after the plant is twelve inches tall. To harvest just the leaves, cut them above the bulbous part of the stem. When harvesting the bottom of the stems, which look like fat scallions, pull off dried leaves until you get to the white center. Soak them in water because, like leeks, gritty dirt can get down in between the leaf layers. Both leaves and stems can be dried or frozen for storage.

How to Use the Herb

Lemongrass shares many insect-repelling compounds with its cousin citronella (*Cymbopogon nardus*) and has been used to repel fleas, ticks, and lice. While outside, just crush a leaf and rub it on your skin. In advance of an outing, make a cream that you can apply at home or take with you. The cream or a bath infusion can be used as treatment for ringworm. In addition, a bath infusion helps get rid of scabies and head lice. Lemongrass can be combined with bay for soothing insect bites and stings. An infusion can be dabbed on affected areas or used to make a cream.

TAKE THE STING OUT OF BITES LEMONGRASS INFUSION

3 tablespoons dried lemongrass leaves, crumbled

1 tablespoon dried lavender flowers, crumbled

1 teaspoon dried chamomile flowers, crumbled

1 teaspoon dried peppermint leaves, crumbled

1 cup boiling water

Combine the herbs and then add the water. Steep for 30 to 60 minutes and strain.

The fungicidal properties of lemongrass make it an effective treatment for athlete's foot, vaginitis, and jock itch. The Lemongrass and Lavender Tea helps deal with these issues internally and topically while it also provides stress relief. Drink one to four cups of tea a day.

LEMONGRASS AND LAVENDER TEA

2 teaspoons dried lemongrass leaves, crumbled

2 teaspoons dried lavender flowers, crumbled

2 cups boiling water

Combine the herbs and add the water. Steep for 10 to 20 minutes and strain.

The tea or a stronger infusion can be used for a compress to place on affected areas, or it can be used for a foot soak or sitz bath. Fresh lemongrass can be used to make a poultice, too. In addition, the poultice or a bath with a lemongrass infusion is effective in easing arthritis pain.

Lemongrass has strong antiseptic properties that make it ideal for treating sore throats and laryngitis. Brew a tea with 2 teaspoons of lemongrass in 1 cup of water and use it as a gargle or mouthwash. The tea can also be used to reduce a fever.

The same properties that make it good to treat sore throats also make it an ideal astringent for toning the skin and treating acne. Use the tea at room temperature, or in the summer chill it in the fridge before splashing it on your face.

Like many herbs, lemongrass supports a healthy digestive tract and can be used to relieve digestive problems such as stomach pain, indigestion, gastroenteritis, and flatulence. Make a tea with 1 or 2 teaspoons of dried leaves in 1 cup of boiling water. Steep for ten to fifteen minutes. Drink a cup once or twice a day. If you prefer a tincture instead of tea, take ½ to 1 teaspoon once or twice a day.

The bulbous bottom of the lemongrass stem is used in Asian cooking and is a common ingredient in Thai food. Try it in a vegetable stir-fry or any dish that can be enhanced with a lemony taste without the sourness of lemon. Because it combines well with garlic and chili peppers, lemongrass enhances the flavor of salsa.

Salsa with a Lemony Lemongrass Twist

2 stalks lemongrass, cut into a few large pieces

6 medium tomatoes, diced

1 chili pepper (or more if you like it hot), diced

1 onion, diced

1 garlic clove, pressed

2 tablespoons cilantro, chopped

1 tablespoon olive oil

Place the tomatoes in a blender or food processor and give it a few pulses. Add the onion, chili pepper, garlic, and olive oil, and pulse again a few times. Pour the mixture into a bowl, add the cilantro and lemongrass, and mix well. Let it sit in the fridge for an hour or two. Remove the lemongrass, stir, and serve.

....

A medicinal honey made with lemongrass leaves will add a nice lemony flavor to tea as it aids the digestive system. Also, freeze chopped leaves into ice cube trays to flavor summer drinks.

How to Use the Essential Oils

The color of lemongrass essential oil can be yellow, amber, or reddish-brown. It has a fresh, grassy citrus scent with earthy undertones.

Lemongrass helps ease arthritic joint pain, rheumatism, general muscle pain, nerve pain, and sprains. Combine it with lavender and rosemary to boost its effects.

LEMONGRASS PAIN RELIEVER MASSAGE BLEND

5 drops lemongrass essential oil

4 drops lavender essential oil

3 drops rosemary essential oil

1 ounce carrier oil

Mix the essential oils together and then combine with the carrier oil. Coconut works well as a carrier oil.

....

Use lemongrass on its own or blend it with lavender and chamomile to relieve headaches, mental fatigue, nervous exhaustion, and stress. This mix works nicely in a diffuser, too. For headaches, dilute the blend to 1 percent to massage the temples. Do this by doubling the amount of carrier oil or by using half the amount of essential oils.

Lemongrass, lavender, and peppermint make an effective insect repellent blend that can be used for an ointment or a cream. This combination of oils can also be used to scent the air and keep insects out of the house or away from a patio area while dining. Cut foot-long strips of cotton ribbons, dip them in the essential oil blend (there is no need to use a carrier oil for this), and then hang them in open windows or around your patio. Use red, white, and blue ribbons for Fourth of July celebrations or any colors that suit the occasion. If ribbons aren't your thing, use the blend in a diffuser or vaporizer.

Marjoram

(Origanum majorana L., syn. *Majorana hortensis)*

Also known as: Joy of the Mountain, Knotted Marjoram, Sweet Marjoram

Marjoram shares the common name, Joy of the Mountain, with its close cousin oregano (*Origanum vulgare*). The name marjoram can be confusing because oregano has the common name of Wild Marjoram. In addition, *Thymus mastichina*, a type of thyme, is also called Wild Marjoram.[38]

Considered a sweeter version of oregano, marjoram was used by the ancient Greeks to treat rheumatism and by the Romans for indigestion. Water scented with marjoram was used for bathing and for laundry. During the Middle Ages it was more popular than thyme in Britain, perhaps because both John Gerard and Nicholas Culpeper sang its praises in their herbals.

Marjoram was used as a general strewing herb and for fumigating sickrooms. In Elizabethan England, marjoram, rosemary, and sage were mixed with wine to treat blackened teeth. Not wanting to leave it behind, early European settlers brought it with them and introduced the plant into North America. Marjoram has been used to create various green dyes.

Medicinal Uses

Anxiety, appetite stimulant, arthritis, asthma, bronchitis, bruises, carpal tunnel, catarrh, chest congestion, chilblains, chronic fatigue, colds, constipation, cough, digestive system support, flatulence, flu, hay fever, headache, heartburn, indigestion, insomnia, joint stiffness, menstrual cramps, menstrual cycle problems, migraine, motion sickness, muscle ache or pain, muscle strain, nasal congestion, nausea, nervous system support, premenstrual syndrome (PMS), rheumatism, sciatica, sinusitis, sore throat, sprains, temporomandibular joint pain (TMJ), upset stomach

Precautions and Contraindications

The herb: Do not use medicinally during pregnancy.

The essential oils: Avoid during pregnancy; use in moderation; may cause drowsiness.

Parts of Plant Used

Herbal remedies: Leaves and flowers

Essential oils: Leaves, flowers, and buds

Culinary purposes: Leaves

---

38. Jeanne Rose, *375 Essential Oils and Hydrosols* (Berkeley, CA: Frog, Ltd., 1999), 150.

Growing and Harvesting

Marjoram grows about twelve inches tall and has the hallmark square stems of the mint family. The stems are angular with numerous branches, giving the plant a bushy appearance. The small, oval leaves are gray-green and slightly fuzzy. The green buds look like knots until they open into spherical clusters of tiny white or pink flowers. They bloom from late summer to early autumn.

Type	Zone	Light	Soil	Moisture	Height	Spacing
Perennial	9	Full sun	Sandy	Moderately dry	12"	6–8"

Because the seeds are slow to germinate and the seedlings are so tiny, it is generally easier to purchase plants. While it prefers full sun, marjoram can tolerate partial shade. Marjoram is a tender perennial that is frequently grown as an annual in cooler zones, however, in warm climates it is possible to get two harvests in a season. It does well as a houseplant. Although marjoram can be propagated by sowing fresh seeds, root division or stem cuttings are easier. The roots can become aggressive if not divided regularly every few years.

Marjoram is a good companion to asparagus, beets, cucumbers, lettuce, onions, peas, potatoes, squash, corn, tomatoes, sage, and zucchini. It improves the growth and flavor of most plants growing nearby. Marjoram repels ants.

The leaves can be harvested anytime after the plant is seven or eight inches tall. They will retain flavor, color, and potency when dried. The plant can be cut back to the first set of leaves to encourage new growth.

How to Use the Herb

We will see why the famous English herbalists touted the merits of this plant. Like most members of the mint family, marjoram is an aid for easing and treating digestive issues. Not only does it improve digestion, marjoram also stimulates the appetite, relieves indigestion and heartburn, and soothes an upset stomach. In addition, it reduces flatulence and alleviates constipation. Use a tea or infusion of marjoram to settle the stomach and counteract nausea or motion sickness. Drink up to three cups of marjoram tea a day while treating a particular problem.

Marjoram Digestive Rescue Tea

1–2 teaspoons dried flowers and leaves, crumbled

1 cup boiling water

Pour the water over the herbs. Steep for 10 to 15 minutes and strain.

As an alternative to the digestive tea, use one half to one teaspoon of tincture three times a day. Marjoram can be combined with anise and lemon balm for a tea that settles upset stomach. Instead of a full cup, drink a little at a time.

SETTLE THE TUMMY MARJORAM TEA

2 teaspoons dried marjoram flowers and leaves, crumbled

½ teaspoon anise seeds, crushed

½ teaspoon dried lemon balm leaves, crumbled

2 cups boiling water

Pour the water over the herbs. Steep for 10 to 15 minutes and strain.

....

The antibacterial and antiviral properties of marjoram make it a good herb to use during cold and flu season. It soothes catarrh and disinfects the inflamed mucous membranes. A tea, infusion, or tincture can be used to ease respiratory problems related to asthma, bronchitis, hay fever, colds, and sinusitis. The tea is helpful to calm a tickly cough and can be used as a gargle to soothe a sore throat. Also try a tea using marjoram, thyme, and lavender in equal amounts to drink or to make a warm compress for the chest. A steam inhalation using equal amounts of marjoram and peppermint is another good way to treat congestion and respiratory problems.

Marjoram can be worked into the diet as it goes well with other herbs such as thyme, basil, and parsley for pasta dishes. It can be sprinkled on meats and poultry for roasting, and used to flavor soups and stews.

Marjoram is a gentle, calming herb that can be used as a sedative and tonic for the nerves. Drink two or three cups of marjoram tea throughout the day to ease anxiety, or have a cup about an hour before bed if insomnia is a problem. As an alternative, a tincture can be taken for anxiety and insomnia as well as to alleviate a tension headache or migraine. Marjoram can also reduce some symptoms of chronic fatigue such as muscle ache and headache.

RELAX AND RELIEVE TENSION MARJORAM TEA

1 teaspoon dried marjoram flowers and leaves, crumbled

½ teaspoon dried chamomile flowers, crumbled

½ teaspoon dried lavender flowers, crumbled

1 cup boiling water

Pour the water over the herbs. Steep for 10 to 15 minutes and strain.

....

The Relax and Relieve Tension Tea can help you fall asleep as well as ease a headache. Increase the amount of herbs to brew an infusion for a relaxing soak in the tub that will also reduce muscle aches and pains.

The antispasmodic properties of marjoram make it helpful in relieving menstrual cramps and for stimulating menstrual flow. It also eases the symptoms of PMS.

How to Use the Essential Oils

The color of marjoram essential oil ranges from pale yellow to amber. It has a spicy herbaceous scent with a slightly woody undertone.

An infusion of the herb or essential oil can be used for an effective massage oil to ease muscle aches, pains, and strains. This warming herb aids in increasing joint flexibility to relieve arthritis and rheumatism. Marjoram's anti-inflammatory properties also help relieve carpal tunnel pain, sciatica, and temporomandibular joint pain (TMJ). Use half the amount of essential oil as listed for the Muscle Warming Massage recipe when applying to the face to relieve TMJ, as facial skin is more sensitive.

MARJORAM MUSCLE WARMING MASSAGE OIL

7 drops marjoram essential oil

3 drops rosemary essential oil

2 drops lemongrass essential oil

1 ounce carrier oil

Mix the essential oils together and then combine with the carrier oil.

....

Marjoram can be used to treat sprains and strains or to soothe tired or stiff muscles after sports or any kind of overexertion. Make a warm compress with 2 drops of chamomile and 1 drop of marjoram in 1 quart of water. Of course, soaking in the tub is another way to relax overworked muscles or to just warm up on a winter's night.

WARMING WINTER BATH WITH MARJORAM

5 drops rosemary essential oil

4 drops marjoram essential oil

3 drops lavender essential oil

1 ounce carrier oil

or 2 cups Epsom or sea salts

For bath oil, combine the essential oils, then add to the carrier oil. When making bath salts, mix the essential oils together. Place the salts in a glass bowl, add the essential oils, and mix thoroughly. Store in a jar with a tight lid.

....

Marjoram essential oil is effective with apricot kernel or jojoba carrier oils to treat chilblains and bruises. Also, the essential oil can be used in a diffuser or as a steam inhalation to ease respiratory problems related to asthma, bronchitis, and colds.

The Mints

Peppermint (*Mentha x piperita*)

Also known as: Balm Mint, Brandy Mint

Spearmint (*Mentha spicata* L., syn. *M. viridis*)

Also known as: Green Mint, Lamb Mint, Our Lady's Mint, Sage of Bethlehem

Peppermint is a naturally-occurring hybrid between spearmint and water mint (*Mentha aquatica*). Its species name comes from the Latin *piper*, "pepper," because the taste of this herb has a hint of pepper. While spearmint is considered the oldest species of mint, peppermint has been around for quite a long time, too. Dried peppermint leaves have been found in Egyptian burials dating to 1000 BCE.

The Greeks and Romans valued both mints for help with digestive issues. Spearmint leaves were sprinkled in bath water for restorative soaks by the Greeks. Both mints were introduced into England by the Romans. By the eighteenth century, peppermint and spearmint were widely used for medicinal and culinary purposes throughout Europe and North America.

Spearmint is the most commonly grown culinary mint. It is milder and less pungent than peppermint. Spearmint is sweet, whereas peppermint has a sharp flavor. In addition, it is second only to peppermint as a healing mint. Peppermint is so effective for many applications because it contains menthol; spearmint does not.

Medicinal Uses

Peppermint: Acne, asthma, bad breath, belching, bronchitis, burns, chest congestion, chilblains, colds, cough, dermatitis, diarrhea, digestive system support, expectorant, flatulence, flu, gallstones, gingivitis, gout, headache, heartburn, indigestion, infection, inflammation, insect bites and stings, insect repellent, irritable bowel syndrome (IBS), motion sickness, muscle ache or pain, muscle strains, nasal congestion, nausea, nerve pain, nervous system support, rashes, scabies, skin care, sleep aid, sore throat, sprains, stomachache or pain, stomach ulcer, sunburn, tonsillitis, tooth decay, upset stomach

Spearmint: Acne, anxiety, appetite stimulant, bad breath, belching, burns, chest congestion, colds, cough, digestive system support, flatulence, gallstones, gingivitis, heartburn, hyperactivity, indigestion, motion sickness, muscle ache or pain, nasal congestion, nausea, nerve pain, nervous system support, scabies, skin care, sleep aid, sore throat, tooth decay, upset stomach

Precautions and Contraindications

The peppermint herb: Avoid with high blood pressure; do not use when pregnant or nursing; not compatible with homeopathic treatments; use in moderation; do not give to children under five; avoid with hiatal hernia or acute gallstones.

The peppermint essential oils: Avoid with high blood pressure; may cause skin irritation in some; should not be used on children under twelve.

The spearmint essential oils: May cause dermatitis in some; may cause sensitivity, especially in children.

Parts of Plants Used

Herbal remedies for both mints: Mainly leaves, sometimes the flowers

Essential oils for both mints: Leaves, flowers, and buds

Culinary purposes for both mints: Leaves

Growing and Harvesting

Both mints have the distinctive feature of square stems. Peppermint reaches twelve to thirty-six inches in height. Its dark green leaves are deeply veined and toothed. Tiny purple, pink, or white flowers grow in whorls at the tops of the stems. It blooms from midsummer to early autumn.

Spearmint has tight whorls of pink or lilac-colored flowers atop spikes of bright green leaves. Like peppermint, its leaves are deeply veined and toothed. It reaches twelve to eighteen inches tall and blooms from late summer to early autumn.

Herb	Type	Zone	Light	Soil	Moisture	Height	Spacing
Peppermint	Perennial	5	Full sun to partial shade	Loam or slight clay	Moist	12–36"	12–24"
Spearmint	Perennial	4	Partial shade	Loam	Moist	12–18"	12–24"

Mints are a mainstay of many gardens, perhaps because they are hardy and easy to grow in average soil. However, you have to keep an eye on these plants because, with creeping roots, mints can be extremely invasive. Mints are good candidates for containers or they can be kept in check with barriers sunk into the ground around their roots. In addition, keep different types of mint in different beds or containers because they hybridize easily. The resulting herbs will not taste as good as their parent plants or be medicinally potent.

Both mints repel white cabbage moths, aphids, flea beetles, and ants. Peppermint also repels bees. They both attract hoverflies and predatory wasps, and are good companions to cabbages and tomatoes. In addition, peppermint is a good companion to cayenne and chamomile. Neither mint is a good companion to parsley. Rodents don't like mints and can be repelled by strewing an area with fresh leaves. Peppermint and spearmint can be propagated by root division, stem cuttings, or layering.

Leaves can be harvested when plants reach six to eight inches tall. The plants can be cut back to encourage a second crop. The leaves of both mints dry well, however, peppermint holds its fragrance and flavor better than spearmint. Remove the leaves from the stems and screen dry. Both mints also freeze well.

How to Use the Herb

Most members of the mint family of herbs are well known for quelling a range of digestive issues. Peppermint and spearmint can be considered king and queen of the mints. Even though it is milder, spearmint is as good as peppermint for many digestive issues. Because peppermint tea can be too strong for children, spearmint is a better choice.

Both mints are anesthetic stomach soothers, relieving upset stomach, flatulence, heartburn, belching, and indigestion. Because they ease nausea, they are effective for motion sickness. In addition, they are both helpful in the treatment of gallstones. A tea made with either mint is an effective mouthwash for bad breath as it prevents gingivitis and tooth decay. Spearmint can be used to stimulate the appetite, and as a tea it makes a good rinse to clear the mouth when sick or a gargle for sore throat. It also works well in other teas to flavor herbs that are less tasty. Both mints aid in keeping the digestive tract healthy. Adding a little honey to mint tea for taste will also help soothe indigestion.

DIGESTIVE MINT TEA
2 teaspoons dried peppermint, crumbled
or 3 teaspoons dried spearmint, crumbled
or 1½ teaspoons of either, crumbled
1 cup boiling water

When making tea, let the water come down from the boiling point. This is especially important when using spearmint because it is more heat sensitive. Steep for 10 minutes and strain.

As an alternative to the digestive tea, mix either mint in equal amounts with chamomile flowers and dill leaves. For mild nausea, just add mint leaves to a glass of water or lemonade.

Peppermint relieves stomach pain and diarrhea and reduces inflammation of stomach ulcers and gout. It also balances intestinal flora and relieves IBS. Instead of a tea or infusion, a tincture can be used for digestive problems and capsules for IBS.

Both mints soothe the nerves, and either one with chamomile works as a sleep aid. Spearmint can be used in equal amounts with chamomile but if you make it with peppermint, use less of it than chamomile. A mild spearmint tea with lemon balm can help calm a child's anxiety or hyperactivity, while a strong peppermint tea is good for an adult's after-lunch perk-up in place of coffee. Drink one or two cups a day of the Calming Spearmint Infusion for a day or two to ease anxiety.

Calming Spearmint Infusion

3 tablespoons dried spearmint leaves, crumbled

2 tablespoons dried chamomile flowers, crumbled

1 tablespoon dried lemon balm leaves, crumbled

1 quart of water

Combine the herbs and then add the water. Steep for 30 to 60 minutes and strain.

....

The menthol content of peppermint makes it ideal for treating colds, flu, nasal and chest congestion, coughs, sore throat, and tonsillitis. Also, the nutrients in peppermint are helpful during sickness. This herb is very effective as a steam inhalation that clears the sinuses and helps soothe asthma and bronchitis. The tea also works as an expectorant.

Soothe and Heal Peppermint Tea

1 teaspoon dried peppermint, crumbled

½ teaspoon dried rosemary, crumbled

½ teaspoon dried thyme, crumbled

Combine the herbs and then add the water. Steep 10 to 15 minutes and strain. Add a little honey to taste.

....

Brew an infusion of the same three herbs—peppermint, rosemary, and thyme—to make a chest rub for additional relief. Although milder, spearmint can be used to treat colds, coughs, chest and nasal congestion, and sore throat.

The mints are great for the complexion, too. Peppermint fights the bacterial infection of acne and stimulates circulation for a good complexion. In its own right, spearmint is an astringent that heals complexion blemishes and is a better choice for those of us with sensitive skin.

Minty Face Wash

1 cup fresh peppermint, chopped

or 1 cup fresh spearmint leaves, chopped

1 quart cool water

Allow the leaves to soak for about an hour, strain.

....

The face wash is especially nice on a hot summer day. A spearmint wash helps heal chapped hands in the winter or any time of year. An ointment made with a peppermint infusion relieves the itching of dermatitis and sunburn.

Brew an infusion with either mint for a bath to kill scabies mites. As an alternative, combine either mint with lavender or thyme in any percentage for this purpose. Use a quart of a strong infusion in the tub.

In the summer, hang a few bunches of either mint to cool and freshen a room. This is also a good way to freshen a sickroom.

How to Use the Essential Oils

The peppermint essential oil is clear to pale yellow or greenish with a strong minty, camphoraceous scent. The spearmint oil is clear to pale yellow, to olive with a spicy, herbaceous, minty scent. It is less pungent than peppermint.

An ointment made with peppermint essential oil can be used as an insect repellent that also soothes the swelling and itching of bites. It can be used to relieve skin irritation, rashes, and chilblains, too. Also, for easing and healing minor burns add 1 or 2 drops of either mint to 2 tablespoons of honey.

SKIN SOOTHING PEPPERMINT OINTMENT

¼–½ cup jojoba or beeswax

½–1 cup apricot kernel oil

1 teaspoon peppermint essential oil

Place the jojoba or beeswax in a mason jar in a saucepan of water. Warm over low heat until it begins to melt; add the carrier oil. Stir gently for about 15 minutes. Remove from heat, add the essential oil and stir. Test the thickness by placing a little on a plate and letting it cool in the fridge for a minute or two. If you want it firmer, add more jojoba or beeswax. If it's too thick, add a tiny bit of oil. Let it cool and then store in a cool, dark place.

Both mints ease muscle and nerve pain. Peppermint can be used to reduce inflammation and swelling of sprains and strains. See the profile for rosemary for the Rosemary Warming Massage Oil recipe that includes peppermint. For a headache, mix a drop of peppermint with a teaspoon of carrier oil and use it to massage the temples. To boost the effect, add a drop of lavender.

Parsley

(Petroselinum crispum)

Also known as: Common Parsley, Garden Parsley

Familiar to many as a dinner plate garnish, parsley was commonly used by the Greeks and Romans as a digestive aid and a breath sweetener. Hippocrates, Dioscorides, and Pliny wrote about its properties for treating a range of problems.

During the Middle Ages this herb was used to guard against the plague, and more commonly, a salve made from the seeds was used to treat head lice. Parsley remained popular in Europe through the sixteenth century for a range of culinary and medicinal purposes. In addition, parsley has been used to make green dyes.

This plant's genus name is derived from the Greek *petros*, meaning "rock" or "stone" and refers to its habitat of rocky soil in the Mediterranean region. *Selinon* is the Greek name for wild parsley. [39]

Medicinal Uses

Amenorrhea, anemia, appetite stimulant, arthritis, bad breath, bladder infection, breastfeeding weaning, bruises, dandruff, digestive system support, eye problems, flatulence, gout, hair care, hay fever, indigestion, inflammation, insect bites and stings, kidney stones, mastitis, menstrual cramps, menstrual cycle problems, premenstrual syndrome (PMS), rheumatism, sciatica

Precautions and Contraindications

The herb: Excessive amounts of the seeds can be toxic; avoid during pregnancy and while nursing; those with kidney disease should avoid.

The essential oils: May irritate the skin in some.

Parts of Plant Used

Herbal remedies: Leaves, roots, and seeds

Essential oils: Seeds

Culinary purposes: Leaves and roots

Growing and Harvesting

Parsley reaches about twelve inches tall and grows in clumps or rounded mounds. Long, erect leaf stems grow from the crown of the plant. The pinnate leaves are deep green and have curly, ruffled edges. Tiny, yellow-green flowers grow in umbels on separate stalks and bloom from midsummer

---

39. Jeanne D'Andrea, *Ancient Herbs in the J. Paul Getty Museum Gardens* (Malibu, CA: J. Paul Getty Museum, 1989), 68.

to autumn in the second year. The gray-brown seeds are oval, ribbed, and approximately an eighth of an inch long. The white root looks like a small carrot.

Type	Zone	Light	Soil	Moisture	Height	Spacing
Biennial	5	Full sun to partial shade	Loam	Moist	12"	8–10"

Parsley does well in average garden soil but does even better when it is well composted. It is at home in a container on a porch or in the house on a sunny windowsill. It also makes a nice addition to hanging baskets. Parsley is propagated by sowing fresh seeds, however, they are very slow to germinate. This herb is a good companion to most vegetables, but it does not like being planted next to any type of mint. Although parsley is a biennial, it is best grown as an annual as it does not produce many leaves in the second year.

Leaves can be harvested after the plant has at least eight of them, and can be taken from the outer stalks throughout the season. Cut the stems about an inch above the crown of the plant. It can be pruned back to encourage a second harvest. Use a microwave or dehydrator, as parsley leaves lose their flavor and color when air dried. Freezing works well. Harvest the seeds just before they begin to fall.

How to Use the Herb

Often regarded as a decorative garnish and thrown away, this seemingly humble little herb is a nutritional powerhouse and worth working into the diet to maintain good health. It is rich in vitamins, calcium, iron, and other minerals. In addition to being a tonic for wellness, it is good for those with anemia or recovering from illness.

Parsley is also rich in zinc, and is good for men's reproductive health. It goes well with most foods except for sweets. Parsley is part of the *bouquet garni* and *fines herbes* mixtures because it brings out the flavor of other herbs. Chopped parsley can be used to flavor cooking water for pasta or added to soups, stews, veggie dishes, fish, and poultry. When sautéing fish, add several handfuls of parsley leaves to cook along with it. For a warm-up meal on a chilly night, make a potato leek soup that's just a little different.

LEEK AND POTATO SOUP WITH PARSLEY
4 tablespoons butter, margarine, or oil
1 pound potatoes, cubed
1 cup fresh parsley leaves, chopped
or ½ cup dried parsley leaves, crumbled

3 medium sized leeks, sliced

4 cups vegetable broth

4 cups water

Salt and pepper to taste

Melt the butter, add the leeks and sauté for about 3 minutes. Add the water, vegetable broth, and potatoes. Simmer on medium heat for 45 minutes. Mash the potatoes in the pot, add the parsley, salt, and pepper. Stir well and simmer for another 15 to 20 minutes. Serve hot with warm, crusty bread.

....

For other culinary uses, try a parsley-infused oil for cooking or fresh parsley leaves in equal amounts with basil for pesto. Combine equal parts of parsley, rosemary, and sage in red wine vinegar to use on salads or grate fresh parsley root to sprinkle on a salad. Parsley also makes a nice herb butter. As for that decorative garnish, don't throw it away as parsley can remove the smell of onions and garlic from the breath.

For remedies, the root is more effective than the leaves, and the seeds are stronger than the root. In addition to an essential oil, there is also an oil made from pressed parsley seeds, which is very potent and must be used in small amounts.

Parsley is good for almost any urinary tract problem. As a diuretic, it is especially useful for bladder infections because passing more urine helps remove bacteria from the system. This also makes it an aid in treating kidney stones. A decoction made from the root and used for a hot compress can be applied to the bladder or kidney area to help relieve discomfort. In addition, tea made from parsley helps cleanse the blood and rid the body of toxins. When using Flush the System Parsley Tea made with the roots, drink two to three cups a day while treating a condition. When it is made with the seeds, limit your intake to two cups a day.

FLUSH THE SYSTEM PARSLEY TEA

1 teaspoon dried root, chopped

or ½ teaspoon seeds, crushed

1 cup boiling water

When using the root, let it simmer for 10 to 15 minutes, and then let it steep for 10 minutes. When making the tea with seeds, steep for 10 to 15 minutes. Strain before drinking.

....

Parsley is also an aid for gout, arthritis, and rheumatism because it flushes waste from inflamed joints. The diuretic properties that make it effective for urinary tract issues also help alleviate premenstrual bloating and other PMS discomforts. Parsley tea can aid with amenorrhea or help stimulate a late menstrual cycle. It also relieves cramps. Drink two or three cups of tea a day or take a quarter of a teaspoon of tincture four times a day.

Parsley Leaf Tea

1–2 teaspoons dried leaves, crumbled

1 cup boiling water

Pour the water over the leaves and steep for 10 to 15 minutes.

....

Parsley tea helps dry up breast milk after weaning. A poultice of the leaves can be used to treat the discomfort of swollen breasts and mastitis.

The tea can also be used to stimulate the appetite and to treat indigestion and flatulence. Parsley's anti-inflammatory properties inhibit the release of histamine, making this a good herbal tea to drink during hay fever season. Also, use the tea to make a warm compress for the eyes to relieve puffiness.

A poultice made from fresh parsley leaves is effective in relieving bee, mosquito, and wasp stings. When the poultice is used to treat bruises, the discoloration usually subsides in a couple of days. In addition, an infusion of the leaves makes a nice rinse for dark hair to make it shinier. A parsley rinse will also help treat dandruff.

How to Use the Essential Oils

The color of parsley essential oil ranges from yellow to amber. It has a woody spicy, herbaceous scent.

Parsley oil is effective in relieving pain due to its anti-inflammatory properties. Use it for massage to ease arthritis, rheumatism, and sciatica.

Rub the Pain Away Parsley Massage Oil

3 drops coriander essential oil

2 drops parsley essential oil

2 drops clary sage essential oil

1 tablespoon carrier oil

Mix the essential oils together and then combine with the carrier oil.

Peppermint: See the Mints

Rosemary

(Rosmarinus officinalis L.)

Also known as: Compass Plant, Incensier, Rosmarine, Sea Dew

Often found growing on the sea cliffs of southern France, rosemary has been described as having the smell of the ocean with a hint of pine. This is the source of its genus name *Rosmarinus*, which means "dew of the sea." [40] Made with brandy and rosemary as its base, Hungary Water, also known as Queen of Hungary Water, was created in 1370 for Queen Elizabeth of Hungary. While it served as a perfume and a beauty treatment, it also cured her rheumatism.

During the Middle Ages, rosemary blossoms were sugared and eaten as a preventive measure against the plague. At other times, this herb was burned in hospitals to fumigate rooms and clear airborne infections. It was also an important strewing herb that kept homes smelling fresh. Rosemary was one of the ingredients in the classic sixteenth century Eau-de-Cologne, which was used for headaches and as a nerve tonic. Throughout the centuries before refrigeration, it was an important food preservative, especially for meats. In addition, rosemary has been used to create various green dyes.

Medicinal Uses

Acne, arthritis, asthma, athlete's foot, bad breath, bronchitis, burns, cardiovascular system support, chest congestion, colds, cuts and scrapes, dandruff, eczema, fainting, flatulence, flu, hair care, headache, immune system support, indigestion, infection, inflammation, lymph circulation, mental fatigue, migraine, mouth ulcers, muscle ache or pain, muscle strains, nasal congestion, nervous exhaustion, nervous system support, psoriasis, rheumatism, sinusitis, sore throat, sprains, stomachache or pain, stress, temporomandibular joint pain (TMJ), varicose veins

Precautions and Contraindications

The herb: Avoid therapeutic doses during pregnancy; avoid with high blood pressure; too much may irritate the stomach.

The essential oils: Avoid during pregnancy; avoid with epilepsy or other seizure disorders; avoid with high blood pressure; may irritate sensitive skin.

---

40. Wilson, *Aromatherapy*, 113.

Parts of Plant Used

Herbal remedies: Leaves and flowers

Essential oils: Leaves, flowers, and buds

Culinary purposes: Leaves

Growing and Harvesting

Rosemary is a shrubby, evergreen that grows three to six feet tall. Mature stems are woody and brown. Rosemary has short, stiff, needlelike leaves similar to spruce trees. The leaves are dark green on top and pale or white underneath. Pale blue flowers grow in clusters of two or three along the leaf branches. They bloom from late winter to early spring and sometimes intermittently throughout the year.

Type	Zone	Light	Soil	Moisture	Height	Spacing
Perennial	8	Full sun	Sandy	Dry	3–6'	24–36"

Because the seeds are difficult to germinate, it is usually recommended to start with a plant. Rosemary grows slowly in its first year. Also, it does not transplant well, so if you live in a zone where it can be grown outside, plant it in a location where it will stay. It can be propagated by root division and stem cuttings or layering. Rosemary is a companion to sage, beans, and cabbage. It repels snails, slugs, bean beetles, and cabbage flies. It attracts bees.

For those of us who cannot plant it outside, rosemary can be grown in a container. It needs a good sunny window and does not like dry, overheated rooms in the winter. Misting the leaves helps as long as the room has good air circulation because it can develop powdery mildew if it is too humid.

Up to four-inch lengths can be harvested from the branches but never take more than 20 percent of the plant because it does not spring back after a severe cutting as other herbs do. Sprigs freeze well and have a stronger flavor and aroma than fresh. They can also be screen dried or hung.

How to Use the Herb

Most famously, rosemary has been considered a tonic for the brain, improving memory and concentration. Considered a warming herb, it promotes the circulation of blood to the head and the intake of oxygen at the cellular level, which improves brain function. Rosemary helps to normalize low blood pressure and contributes to a heart-healthy diet. This herb also improves lymph and blood circulation. Because of increased blood flow, it aids in relieving headaches and migraines.

GET THE BLOOD GOING ROSEMARY TEA

1–2 teaspoons dried rosemary leaves, crumbled

1 cup boiling water

Pour the water over the leaves. Steep for 10 to 15 minutes and strain.

....

As an alternative, use equal amounts of rosemary and peppermint in the Get the Blood Going Rosemary Tea for an invigorating lift. Tea made with just rosemary can be used for a compress to relieve headaches, too. For a migraine make an infusion and take two to three tablespoons every three hours. The tea and infusion also serve as a tonic for the nerves, and helps cope with mental fatigue and nervous exhaustion. Additionally, half a teaspoon of rosemary tincture once a day is a tonic for stress.

As a pungent aromatic, rosemary clears nasal and chest congestion due to colds, the flu, or sinusitis. Its antibacterial and antiviral properties fight infection while providing support for the immune system. Used as a steam inhalation, it will soothe inflammation. Rosemary is also an aid for asthma and bronchitis. The leaves, or both flowers and leaves, can be used for these purposes. The physically warming effect and the aromatic vapors of the herbs in the Rosemary Chest Rub Infusion and Ointment work together to provide relief and healing.

ROSEMARY CHEST RUB INFUSION AND OINTMENT

Ingredients for the infusion

2 teaspoons dried rosemary leaves, crumbled

1 teaspoon dried sage leaves, crumbled

1 teaspoon dried thyme leaves, crumbled

1 cup oil

Ingredients for the ointment

¼–½ cup beeswax or jojoba

1 cup infused oil

First, make an infusion by combining the herbs and oil in a double boiler. On very low heat, simmer for 30 to 60 minutes. Remove from heat and let cool. Use a stainless steel strainer lined with cheesecloth over a bowl to strain. Fold the cheesecloth over the herbs to press out as much oil as possible.

To make the ointment, place the jojoba or beeswax in a mason jar in a saucepan of water. Warm over low heat until it begins to melt; add the infused oil. Stir gently with a fork for about 15 minutes. Let it cool. Cover and store in a cool, dark place.

....

The antiseptic properties of rosemary make it a good gargle to soothe a sore throat and to ease mouth ulcers. It also reduces inflammation and helps firm the gums while it fights bad breath. Use 2 teaspoons of dried leaves in 1 cup of water, and steep for thirty minutes. Drink half a cup and use the other half as a mouthwash and gargle.

As a powerful fungicide, rosemary is ideal for treating athlete's foot. Make a hot oil infusion to rub on the skin or to use as a foot soak. A rosemary infusion soothes the itching and inflammation of eczema and psoriasis, too. It also heals burns and cuts, and because it fights bacteria, rosemary helps clear acne. Combine rosemary with lavender and thyme to make an infusion to dab on affected areas, or use the infusion to make a healing cream.

SKIN HEALING ROSEMARY INFUSION

2 teaspoons dried rosemary leaves, crumbled

1 teaspoon dried lavender flowers, crumbled

1 teaspoon dried thyme leaves, crumbled

1 cup boiling water

Combine the herbs and then add the water. Steep for 30 to 45 minutes and strain.

An infusion of rosemary massaged into the scalp promotes hair growth and gets rid of dandruff. Also, steep a fresh sprig or two in a cup of boiling water for about fifteen minutes. When it cools use it as a rinse for brown hair to bring out the highlights.

Not only does rosemary go well with a wide range of food, it also aids digestion by enhancing food absorption. However, when things go awry, brew a cup of rosemary tea or take two ounces of an infusion to relieve indigestion, gas, or stomach pain.

How to Use the Essential Oils

Rosemary essential oil ranges from colorless to pale yellow. Its fresh, herbaceous scent has a woody undertone.

While students in ancient Greece wore a sprig of rosemary in the hair to aid their memory and learning, we can use the essential oil in a diffuser to improve concentration. Using it this way will also help when recovering from stress or chronic illness. In addition, it helps to alleviate headaches.

The steam inhalation mentioned above can be made using essential oil, either rosemary alone or with sage and thyme. Just swish 4 drops of essential oil into 1 quart of steaming water. If you are using a blend, use 2 drops of rosemary and 1 each of sage and thyme.

The warming effects of rosemary work well to relieve the pain and stiffness of rheumatism brought on by cold weather. Massaging with rosemary also relieves the pain and swelling of arthritis, muscle pain or strain, and ligament sprains. Combining rosemary with peppermint and chamomile creates an effective massage oil that also reduces stress.

ROSEMARY WARMING MASSAGE OIL

6 drops rosemary essential oil

4 drops chamomile essential oil

3 drops peppermint essential oil

1 ounce carrier oil

Mix the essential oils together and then combine with the carrier oil.

....

For leg cramps, use 4 drops of rosemary and 2 drops of chamomile in 1 tablespoon of carrier oil to massage away the pain. This will also reduce the appearance of varicose veins and broken capillaries. To treat temporomandibular joint pain (TMJ), use 1 drop of rosemary essential oil in 1 teaspoon of carrier oil. A drop or two of essential oil on a tissue or a handful of crushed sprigs are effective in reviving someone who has fainted.

The Sages

Clary *(Salvia sclarea L.)*

Also known as: Clary Sage, Clary Wort, Clear Eye, Muscatel Sage, See Bright

Sage *(Salvia officinalis L.)*

Also known as: Common Sage, Dalmatian Sage, European Sage, Garden Sage, True Sage

The genus name, *Salvia*, comes from the Latin *salvare*, meaning "to cure" or "make healthy." [41] Clary's species name comes from the Latin *clarus*, meaning "clear." [42] For centuries, clary was used to treat eye problems, which earned it the name Clear Eye. In Germany, it was occasionally substituted for hops to brew certain beers and ales. Clary was also used in muscatel wine.

Considered more for medicinal than culinary purposes, sage has a long history of use by the ancient Egyptians, Greeks, and Romans. It was used throughout Europe and from the sixteenth century onward it was an important herb in British apothecaries. Among other things, sage was considered good for the brain and nervous system. Trade with Asia brought sage to popular use in China, and in the seventeenth century it was introduced into North America. Both clary and sage have been used to create various green and yellow dyes.

Medicinal Uses

Clary: Acne, amenorrhea, asthma, boils, cough, dandruff, eczema, flatulence, hair care, headache, indigestion, laryngitis, menopausal discomforts, menstrual cramps, migraine, muscle aches and pains, nervous tension, premenstrual syndrome (PMS), psoriasis, skin care, sore throat, stomachache or pain, stress, tonsillitis

Sage: Acne, amenorrhea, arthritis, asthma, bad breath, boils, breastfeeding weaning, carpal tunnel, colds, cough, cuts and scrapes, dandruff, diarrhea, digestive system support, eczema, flatulence, flu, gingivitis, headache, indigestion, inflammation, insect bites and stings, laryngitis, menopausal discomforts, menstrual cramps, mouth ulcers, muscle aches and pains, psoriasis, rheumatism, skin care, sore throat, stomachache or pain, tonsillitis, vaginal yeast infection (vaginitis)

Precautions and Contraindications

The clary herb and essential oils: Avoid during pregnancy and while nursing; avoid when taking sedatives or barbiturates.

---

41. Wilson, *Aromatherapy*, 130.
42. Ibid., 61.

The sage herb and essential oils: Should not be used on a daily basis; use in moderation; avoid during pregnancy and while nursing; avoid with epilepsy or other seizure disorders; it should not be used more than three weeks in a row without at least one week break; avoid with high blood pressure or diabetes.

Parts of Plants Used

Clary herbal remedies and essential oils: Leaves and flowering tops

Sage herbal remedies and essential oils: Leaves

Clary and sage culinary purposes: Leaves

Growing and Harvesting

Clary has broad, oblong leaves that are toothed and wrinkled. They are downy underneath. Whorls of small white and lilac or pink flowers grow on leafy spikes and bloom early to midsummer. Reaching two or three feet tall, clary has square, downy stems that range from light green to brown.

Sage grows one to three feet tall and has square, woody base stems covered in down. This plant tends to get bushy and sprawl. Its oblong leaves are light gray-green, wrinkled, and puckered. Leafy stalks bear whorls of small blue-purple flowers that bloom early to midsummer.

Herb	Type	Zone	Light	Soil	Moisture	Height	Spacing
Clary	Biennial	4	Full sun	Slightly sandy loam	Moderately moist	2–3'	9–12"
Sage	Perennial	4	Full sun to partial shade	Sandy loam	Moderately moist	1–3'	24"

While clary prefers moderate moisture, it can also grow in dry conditions. With the right moisture and composting, it will flourish. The flower stalks tend to bend over when they get heavy. Clary attracts bees and sometimes hummingbirds. It can be propagated by sowing fresh seeds or let it help you as it readily self-sows. The leaves can be harvested as needed for fresh use or whole stalks with flowers can be hung or screen dried.

Sage does best in full sun but will tolerate light shade. It needs good spacing because it tends to sprawl. It also does well indoors as long as it gets plenty of sun. Sage can be propagated by stem cuttings or layering, root division, and sowing fresh seeds. While sage is a good companion to beans, cabbage, carrots, strawberries, tomatoes, marjoram, and rosemary, it has a negative effect on onions. This herb repels cabbage loopers, carrot rust flies, and imported cabbage moths. It attracts bees and butterflies. Sage leaves can be harvested as needed for fresh use throughout the season.

Spread the leaves on a screen or hang the stems in very small bundles to air dry. In large bundles, the leaves dry slowly and tend to get a musty odor.

How to Use the Herbs

Don't wait until Thanksgiving to get the sage out of the cupboard because cold and flu season starts in October and this herb can help. Sage aids in preventing colds by simply using it in food, but if illness strikes, sage tea eases cold and flu symptoms. The tea is a nice winter drink that can be boosted with a special winter honey.

SAGE WINTER HONEY

2 tablespoons dried sage, crumbled

2 tablespoons dried thyme, crumbled

2 tablespoons dried rosemary, crumbled

1 tablespoon garlic, chopped

1 cup honey

Pour the honey into a slightly larger jar and set it in a saucepan of water. Warm over low heat until the honey becomes a little less viscous. Add the herbs and garlic and stir with a butter knife to distribute. Continue warming for 15 to 20 minutes, then remove from heat. Put the lid on when cool. Store out of the light at room temperature for a week. Reheat slightly to strain out herbs or leave them in.

Sage tea without honey makes a good mouthwash for bad breath, mouth ulcers, and gingivitis. Alternatively, powdered sage can be gently rubbed on the gums to ease and heal sores and inflammation.

Often considered less important than sage, clary is significant in its own right as a healing herb. A tea made with clary or sage helps ease asthma and coughs. Both of these herbs have antiseptic and astringent properties, making either of them a good choice for treating and soothing sore throats, laryngitis, and tonsillitis. Make a strong tea with the leaves for a gargle. While it is hot, add ½ teaspoon of cider vinegar or 1 teaspoon of salt to ½ cup of tea. Gargle when it is cool enough but still warm.

Like many herbs, sage and clary soothe indigestion and stomach pain, and reduce flatulence. Make a cup of tea or take a teaspoon of tincture. In addition, sage is an aid for digesting meat and for treating mild diarrhea. When treating diarrhea, drink up to three cups a day but not for more than three days.

SAGE DIARRHEA TREATMENT

1–1½ teaspoons dried sage, crumbled

1 cup boiling water

Bring the water to a boil and add the leaves. Simmer for 15 to 20 minutes and strain.

....

When it comes to PMS, clary tea is an uplifting aid to reduce discomfort. Actually, both clary and sage have estrogenlike components that act as mild hormonal stimulants to promote menstruation and treat amenorrhea. A cup of either tea eases menstrual cramps. An infusion can be an aid during menopause, especially for quelling hot flashes. For night sweats, drink a cup of the infusion before going to bed. Additionally, sage can be used to treat vaginal yeast infections. Use a two-fold approach by drinking sage tea and using it as an astringent douche.

The drying properties that make sage good for relieving hot flashes and night sweats, also make it effective to reduce breast milk after weaning. Drink the Post-Weaning Sage Tea three times a day when you are no longer nursing.

POST-WEANING SAGE TEA

½ teaspoon dried sage, crumbled

1 cup boiling water

Pour the water over the herb, steep for 10 to 15 minutes, and strain.

....

Both clary and sage have astringent qualities that make them valuable for treating skin problems including acne, eczema, psoriasis, and boils. An infusion of leaves used for a facial steam is cleansing for the skin and a big help when dealing with acne. An infusion can be used when it is cool for an antiseptic skin wash. It also helps to treat dandruff. Massage the infusion into the scalp after shampooing, then rinse out. Clary is especially effective for oily skin and hair.

Sage relieves insect bites and stings. When you get bitten, just grab a leaf and rub it on the spot. Or make an ointment early in the summer so it's ready to use. Keep it on hand for first-aid treatment of cuts and scrapes, too.

For culinary purposes, clary can be used interchangeably with sage. Its taste is very similar, however, use it sparingly as too much can taste bitter. The warm, pungent flavor of these herbs can perk up so many dishes: omelets, breads, sauces, marinades, any meat or poultry, and a wide range of veggies. Even a grilled cheese sandwich can be jazzed up with a light sprinkling of sage. Also, the combination that has come to be known as the Scarborough Fair herbs (parsley, sage, rosemary, and thyme) goes well on pasta, salads, eggs, and grains.

How to Use the Essential Oils

Clary essential oil is colorless to pale yellow-green. It has a sweet, nutty, herbaceous scent. Sage ranges from colorless to pale yellow. Its scent is spicy warm, herbaceous, and slightly camphoraceous.

While both of these essential oils can be used for treating headaches, clary is the better choice because it is so calming. It helps relieve nervous tension and stress, which can be the underlying cause of a headache. Clary also helps ease migraines. Mix it with lavender and lemon balm for an extra-soothing combination. Use the blend in a diffuser or dilute it to a 1 percent ratio with a carrier oil and dab it on your wrists or rub your temples with it.

CLARY HEADACHE RELIEF DIFFUSER BLEND

6 drops clary essential oil

3 drops lavender essential oil

2 drops lemon balm essential oil

Combine the oils and let the blend mature for about 1 week.

Both clary and sage are effective for relieving muscle aches and pains. However, sage is especially good for treating arthritis, rheumatism, and carpal tunnel pain.

SAGE MUSCLE RUB OIL

6 drops sage essential oil

4 drops rosemary essential oil

2 drops coriander essential oil

1 ounce carrier oil

Mix the essential oils together and then combine with the carrier oil.

St. John's Wort

(Hypericum perforatum L.)

Also known as: Goatweed, Rosin Rose, Sweet Amber

Although considered a weed by some, St. John's wort has a long history in folk medicine. It was popular with the ancient Greeks and Romans for healing and good health. Hippocrates, Pliny, and Dioscorides mentioned it in their writings. The Greeks used it to treat sciatica and other issues of the nervous system. From Roman times through the Crusades, it was used for treating wounds. In the Middle Ages, it was used for a range of ailments. Gerard and other herbalists highly recommended this herb. In addition, St. John's wort has been used to create various red and yellow dyes.

Named because it blooms around the time of St. John's feast day, June 24, its use actually dates to earlier Pagan summer solstice celebrations. The word "wort" comes from the Old English *wyrt,* meaning "plant" or "herb." [43] The name *Rosin Rose* comes from a characteristic of the flowers and buds, which ooze a red liquid that looks like rosin when they are squeezed or bruised.

Medicinal Uses

Anxiety, arthritis, bruises, burns, chicken pox, childbirth, cold sores, cuts and scrapes, dermatitis, eczema, hair care, herpes, infection, inflammation, insect bites and stings, menopausal discomforts, muscle strains, nervous system support, nervous tension, premenstrual syndrome (PMS), psoriasis, rheumatism, scabies, scars, sciatica, seasonal affective disorder (SAD), shingles, skin care, sleep aid, sprains, stress, sunburn, varicose veins

Precautions and Contraindications

The herb: Do not take internally during pregnancy; consult your doctor before using when taking medications.

The infused oils: May cause photosensitivity.

The essential oils: May cause photosensitivity; may cause dermatitis in some.

Parts of Plant Used

Herbal remedies: Leaves, flowers, and buds

Essential oils: Flowers and buds

Culinary purposes: None

---

43. Philip Durkin, *The Oxford Guide to Etymology* (New York: Oxford University Press, 2009), xxxviii.

Growing and Harvesting

St. John's wort is a shrubby plant that reaches two to three feet in height. The round, erect stems have two lengthwise ridges. The pale green leaves are oblong. Bright yellow, star-shaped flowers grow in clusters at the ends of branches. They bloom from mid to late summer and have a light, lemonlike scent. You may find several varieties of St. John's wort plants at garden centers, but *Hypericum perforatum* is the one that is used medicinally.

Type	Zone	Light	Soil	Moisture	Height	Spacing
Perennial	3	Full sun to partial shade	Slightly sandy loam	Moderately dry	2–3'	16–18"

St. John's wort is not a fussy plant. Although it prefers a slightly sandy soil, it does well in average soil. It is easy going about light, too, preferring full sun, however, it does fine in partial shade. St. John's wort can be propagated by root division or by sowing fresh seeds. However, it readily self-sows, which is convenient but you will need to keep an eye on it as it has a tendency to take over the garden.

Harvest leaves before or when the flowers bloom. Use the leaves fresh to make an oil or dry them to store for other uses. Harvest the buds just before opening or when they are slightly opened. To tell if they are ready, give one a gentle squeeze. A reddish-purple liquid will ooze out when it's ready to harvest. Otherwise, give it another day.

How to Use the Herb

St. John's wort became famous when it was reported as a breakthrough treatment for depression. This was followed by reports stating that it did not work, and then more saying that it did. With all the confusion these conflicting reports generated, the many other benefits of this plant were overlooked. On the topic of depression, discuss it with your doctor before using St. John's wort because it can interact with medications.

St. John's wort is effective for dealing with anxiety, nervous tension, stress, and seasonal affective disorder (SAD). It is not an instant cure and usually takes two to three weeks for its effect to become apparent. This herb is restorative for the nervous system. Take one half to one teaspoon of tincture twice a day for a three-week period, stop for one week, and then repeat if necessary.

Lift Me Up St. John's Wort Tincture

6 tablespoons dried St. John's wort leaves, crumbled

3 tablespoons dried lemon balm leaves, crumbled

3 tablespoons dried spearmint leaves, crumbled

1 pint 80 to 100 proof alcohol

Place the herbs in a jar, pour in the alcohol to cover the plant material, close, and shake for 1 to 2 minutes. Set aside for 2 to 4 weeks, shaking the jar every other day. Strain out the herbs and store in a dark glass bottle in a cool, dark place.

....

The same herbs used in the Lift Me Up St. John's Wort Tincture also work well together as a tea to ease PMS and menopausal discomforts. On its own, St. John's wort tea improves the quality of sleep and it is especially soothing with chamomile.

St. John's Wort Ready for Bed Tea

1 teaspoon dried St. John's wort leaves, crumbled

1 teaspoon dried chamomile flowers, crumbled

1 cup boiling water

Combine the herbs and add the water. Steep for 10 to 15 minutes and strain. Add a little honey to taste. Drink the tea 30 minutes to 1 hour before bed.

....

The antiviral and astringent properties of St. John's wort provide relief from cold sores, herpes, chickenpox, and shingles. Drink a cup of tea once a day or take half a teaspoon of tincture in a cup of water two to three times a day. Topically, an infusion of St. John's wort reduces the inflammation of eczema, dermatitis, and psoriasis. Also, use the infused oil or tincture to dab on areas affected by scabies.

If you are outside, crush a flower and rub it on an insect bite or sting to relieve the itching and inflammation. In addition, an infused oil made from the flowers soothes burns and bruises. It relieves pain and promotes tissue repair, and in the case of burns it reduces scarring.

St. John's Wort Soothing Red Oil

¾ cup fresh flowers, leaves, and buds, coarsely chopped

1 pint oil

Place the herbs in a clear glass jar and slowly pour in the oil. Gently swirl the contents to mix. Place the jar where it will stay at room temperature for 2 to 3 weeks. The oil will turn a rich, deep red color. Strain and bottle.

....

Use the infused oil along with olive oil and beeswax to make a salve. During childbirth, the salve is a soothing anti-inflammatory for the perineum. In addition, it will help heal any tears and nerve damage.

Keep the salve on hand in the medicine cabinet as it makes a soothing first-aid dressing for cuts and scrapes. The astringent and antibacterial properties of St. John's wort helps fight infection. The oil or a simple infusion soothes and heals sunburn, too. In addition, a tea made from the flowers and leaves works as a good astringent for oily hair and scalp, and it can be used as a facial toner to improve the complexion.

How to Use the Essential Oils

St. John's wort essential oil ranges from pale yellow to slightly green in color. It has a soft, herbal, balsamic scent.

Like the infused herb, the essential oil can be used topically to relieve the pain and discomfort of cold sores, eczema, dermatitis, and psoriasis. Additionally, it can be used to treat insect bites. Use 1 drop of essential oil in 1 teaspoon of carrier oil. Borage or apricot kernel as the carrier oil will also help to soothe and heal the skin.

To ease the joint and muscle pain of arthritis and rheumatism as well as sciatica, mix 4 to 5 drops of essential oil in 3 teaspoons of carrier oil for massage. This is also effective for gently massaging sprains and strains. In addition, the aromatherapy that goes with the use of this oil will help to reduce stress.

St. John's Wort Sciatica Soak

10 drops St. John's wort essential oil

2 cups sea or Epsom salts

Place the salts in a glass bowl, add the essential oil, and mix well. Store in a jar with a tight lid.

A warm compress using 2 drops of essential oil in 1 quart of hot water works well, too, for joint and muscle pain. To ease the discomfort of varicose veins and aid circulation, do a fomentation of alternating warm and cool compresses. Gently massaging the legs will help relieve the inflammation and swelling of varicose veins.

Spearmint: See the Mints

Thyme
(Thymus vulgaris L.)

Also known as: Common Thyme, English Thyme, Sweet Thyme, White Thyme

Thyme is one of the classic herbs in Mediterranean cuisine that dates back to ancient times. It was used to both flavor food and prevent it from spoiling. The Greeks and Romans not only used this herb in cooking but also as a healing antiseptic. Thyme was an ingredient in a range of remedies and it was used to fumigate homes to avert infectious diseases. Sources differ on whether or not it was the Romans who took it over the Alps into the rest of Europe and Britain. At any rate, it did not take long for this herb to become a universal staple in gardens and medicine chests.

French emperor Charlemagne had thyme planted in all his gardens, and the German abbess Hildegard of Bingen extolled its use for skin problems. In addition to healing remedies, thyme was used as a strewing herb to freshen and disinfect rooms. During World War I it was used as an antiseptic on the battlefield.

Medicinal Uses
Acne, appetite stimulant, arthritis, asthma, athlete's foot, bad breath, bloating, boils, chest congestion, colds, cough, cuts and scrapes, digestive system support, earache, eczema, expectorant, flatulence, flu, gingivitis, hangover, hay fever, headache, immune system support, indigestion, infection, inflammation, menopausal discomforts, menstrual cramps, migraine, muscle ache or pain, nasal congestion, premenstrual syndrome (PMS), psoriasis, scabies, sciatica, sinusitis, skin care, sore throat, sties, stomachache or pain, tonsillitis

Precautions and Contraindications
The herb: Avoid therapeutic doses during pregnancy; avoid with high blood pressure.

The essential oils: Herbal precautions also apply; use in moderation; may cause skin irritation or sensitization in some.

Parts of Plant Used
Herbal remedies: Leaves and flowers

Essential oils: Leaves, flowers, and buds

Culinary purposes: Leaves

Growing and Harvesting

Reaching six to twelve inches tall, thyme is a branching, shrubby herb with woody base stems. The stalkless, lance-shaped leaves are gray-green on top and lighter underneath. The small pink to lilac or bluish-purple flowers grow in little clusters at the ends of the stems. They bloom in midsummer.

Type	Zone	Light	Soil	Moisture	Height	Spacing
Perennial	5	Full sun to partial shade	Sandy loam	Moderately dry	6–12"	10–12"

Thyme does well in sandy to average soil and makes a good edging plant. It grows quite happily in a container by itself or with other herbs. Propagate it by root division and stem cuttings or layering. Thyme is a good companion for eggplants, tomatoes, and potatoes. It repels cabbage worms and whiteflies, and it attracts bees. Additionally, thyme can be used to make an insect spray for your plants. Place a handful of fresh leaves in a large container and pour in 1 quart of boiling water. Let it infuse for a day, strain, and spray on infested plants.

Small amounts of thyme can be harvested throughout the growing season or the entire plant can be cut down to two inches before it blooms. Don't worry, it will grow back and give you a second crop. This herb freezes well or it can be hung or screen dried.

How to Use the Herb

I have to admit that this delightful herb is my favorite for culinary and medicinal purposes. Thyme is one of the Scarborough Fair herbs (parsley, sage, rosemary, and thyme) that go well together in so many foods. Thyme is also one of the herbs in the *bouquets garnis* and *herbes de Provence* classic culinary combinations. Along with oregano and basil, thyme completes a great trio for pasta dishes as well as an herb butter. If you love root vegetables, thyme adds flavor and aids in digesting the starches. Also, infuse thyme with rosemary in olive oil for cooking.

In addition to great taste, this herb fights infection and provides support for the immune system. Classically combined with rosemary for culinary purposes, an infused oil made with these two herbs for cooking during the winter can help prevent colds and flu. Use equal amounts of rosemary and thyme in olive oil.

Thyme aids sluggish digestion, fights gastric and intestinal infections, and stimulates the appetite. It soothes indigestion and relieves stomach pain. A medicinal honey with thyme can be used in after-meal teas to aid digestion and reduce gas or bloating. A simple tea made with thyme works nicely. For variation, use 1 teaspoon of thyme and 1 teaspoon of Roman chamomile, lemon balm, or peppermint.

Thyme to Settle Tea

1–2 teaspoons dried thyme, crumbled

1 cup boiling water

Pour the water over the herb. Steep for 10 minutes and strain.

....

A tincture of thyme can also ease digestive complaints. Take one half to one teaspoon up to three times a day. The antispasmodic properties of thyme that aid digestive problems also make it useful to ease menstrual cramps. The following tea helps to reduce the discomforts of PMS, too. Because thyme contains a number of minerals including iron, it is beneficial at the end of a menstrual period as well as during menopause.

Soothing Thyme Tea for Women

1 teaspoon dried lemon balm leaves, crumbled

½ teaspoon dried thyme leaves, crumbled

½ teaspoon dried marjoram leaves, crumbled

1 cup boiling water

Combine the herbs and pour the water over them. Steep for 10 to 20 minutes and strain.

....

Thyme is useful for a range of respiratory problems including chest colds, wet coughs, hay fever, sinusitis, sore throat, and tonsillitis. Its warming and drying properties aid in clearing congestion. For a respiratory tea, combine equal amounts of thyme and sage. Thyme medicinal honey can soothe the throat and help expel mucus. Brew a tea with just thyme to use as a mouthwash and gargle, which will fight throat infection as well as gingivitis and bad breath. Thyme soothes inflamed mucous membranes and brings relief from asthma attacks. Make a tea with equal amounts of marjoram and lavender to drink or to use for a warm compress for the chest. Not only does this herb fight infection, it also provides support for the immune system.

Like many herbs, thyme eases headaches as well as migraines. Make a mild tea with 1 teaspoon of thyme and 1 cup of water. The tea can also be used for a compress on the temples or neck to relieve a tension headache. Make a stronger infusion to relieve a hangover headache.

Thyme's antibacterial and antifungal properties make it useful in treating boils and sties. Brew a strong tea and carefully dab it on with a cotton swab. Add the tea to a foot soak to relieve athlete's foot. It can also be used to make a warm compress to decrease discomfort and fight infection of an earache. A thyme tincture will disinfect and help heal cuts. Also, try an infusion for the bath to heal irritated or rough skin.

How to Use the Essential Oils

There are a number of thyme essential oils. The one discussed here is called *Thymus vulgaris* CT linalool. This essential oil ranges from clear to pale yellow. It has a herbaceous and slightly sweet scent.

It is important to know a little about thyme essential oils. The first distillation of thyme produces an oil called "red" thyme. This is because the color can be reddish, reddish-brown, or reddish-orange. Distilling the plant material a second time results in white thyme oil, which is clear or pale yellow. Also, the chemical constituents of thyme vary widely according to where it is grown, which is why you will find many types of thyme oils. They are designated with "CT" meaning chemotype. Thyme has about six or seven chemotypes, each with different therapeutic properties. I suggest using *Thymus vulgaris* CT linalool, which is known to be more gentle. Designated as one of the "white" thyme oils, it is often used for people who are sensitive to the stronger types.

During flu season, use the essential oil in a diffuser to disinfect a sickroom. Used as an inhalant, thyme can soothe the inflammation and ease the discomfort of sinus infections. Place a few drops of the essential oil in a clean bottle to use as a nasal inhaler, or increase the potency by mixing it with hyssop and peppermint. Without touching the bottle to your nose, take a couple of deep inhalations. Repeat in a half hour to an hour. The combination of these three herbs, or just thyme on its own, works well as a steam inhalation, too.

CLEAR THE CONGESTION THYME INHALER

2 drops thyme essential oil

2 drops hyssop essential oil

1 drop peppermint essential oil

Combine the oils in a small bottle with a tight lid.

Thyme helps to reduce the inflammation and irritation of acne, eczema, and psoriasis. Mix it with a carrier oil to use on the skin or combine it with lemon balm to make a salve.

HEALING THYME SALVE

½ cup jojoba or beeswax

1 cup sweet almond carrier oil

½ cup borage carrier oil

1 teaspoon lemon balm essential oil

1 teaspoon thyme essential oil

Place the jojoba or beeswax in a mason jar in a saucepan of water. Warm over low heat until it begins to melt; add the carrier oil. Stir gently for about 15 minutes. Remove from heat, add the essential oils and stir. Test the thickness by placing a little on a plate and letting it cool in the fridge for a minute or two. If you want it firmer, add more jojoba or beeswax. If it's too thick, add a tiny bit of oil. Let it cool and then store in a cool, dark place.

....

This herb's anti-inflammatory properties also work well in a massage oil to reduce the muscle and joint pain of arthritis and the discomfort of sciatica. Additionally, try it as a bath soak with sea or Epsom salts.

Thyme can also be used to relieve scabies. Apply it on its own in a carrier oil or mix equal amounts of thyme and lavender and dab it on the affected areas.

Valerian

(Valeriana officinalis L.)

Also known as: Cat Valerian, Common or Garden Valerian, Garden Heliotrope, Vandalroot

Despite the plant's odor, which prompted Greek herbalist Dioscorides to name it *Phu*, valerian was a valued medicinal in the ancient world. It has been used for centuries in Traditional Chinese medicine for a number of ailments. Valerian's common name is thought to have come from the Latin *valere* meaning "to be well." During the Middle Ages it was known as All-heal and Blessed Herb.[44] The name Vandalroot comes from the Swedish *vändelrot*, a reference to its use by Teutonic tribes known as the Vandals.[45] Although the names seem similar, valium does not come from valerian.

Early European settlers brought valerian to North America. Cats and rodents are attracted to this herb, and it is believed that the Pied Piper of Hamelin used valerian to lure the rats away from the city. Cats actually love valerian as much as catnip.

Medicinal Uses

Abdominal pain, anxiety, arthritis, blood pressure, cardiovascular system support, headache, hiccups, hives, indigestion, inflammation, insomnia, menstrual cramps, migraine, muscle ache or pain, muscle strain, nervous system support, nervous tension, restlessness, rheumatism, rheumatoid arthritis, sciatica, sleep aid, stomachache or pain, stress, temporomandibular joint pain (TMJ)

Precautions and Contraindications

The herb: Avoid while pregnant or nursing; avoid if you have liver problems; use in moderation; large doses can cause dizziness, headache, stupor, and vomiting; avoid using for prolonged periods (use for two to three weeks at a time then take a break of at least a week); for some it may stimulate rather than relax.

The essential oils: Herbal precautions also apply; may cause sensitization in some.

Part of Plant Used

Herbal remedies: Roots

Essential oils: Roots

Culinary purposes: None

---

44. Chevallier, *The Encyclopedia of Medicinal Plants*, 146.

45. Arthur O. Tucker and Thomas Debaggio, *The Encyclopedia of Herbs: A Comprehensive Reference to Herbs of Flavor and Fragrance* (Portland, OR: Timber Press, 2009), 498.

Growing and Harvesting

Reaching three to five feet tall, valerian is often regarded as an ornamental plant. Its erect stems are round, hollow, and slightly grooved. The pinnate leaves are dark green and toothed. The small, five-petaled flowers are white with a tinge of pink, however, they can be more pink or even lavender. The flowers grow in dense clusters and bloom from late spring through early to midsummer. The pale brown, clustered root is an upright rhizome with fibrous roots extending outward.

Type	Zone	Light	Soil	Moisture	Height	Spacing
Perennial	4	Partial shade to full sun	Loam	Moist	3–5'	36"

Valerian is easy to grow and does well in a variety of soils, however, a good loam is best. It prefers partial shade but tolerates full sun. If you do not want a lot of it in your garden, remove the flowers before they go to seed as it readily self-sows. Propagate this herb by root division or by letting it self-seed. If you let it reseed, keep an eye on it as it can take over the garden. Valerian attracts butterflies and bees, and it is considered a good companion to most vegetables.

The roots can be harvested in the autumn of the first year or the following spring before new shoots come up. They can be dried in an oven set at 120° Fahrenheit until they are brittle.

How to Use the Herb

Most widely known as a sleep aid and boon for dealing with insomnia, valerian has been called "nature's tranquilizer."[46] In fact, many over-the-counter sleep aids contain valerian. Additionally, people who are trying to reduce and taper off their use of commercial sleeping pills have found valerian helpful. Check with your doctor before using this herb if you take sleeping pills as it can increase the sedative effect of them.

Although the odor has been said to resemble the smell of dirty socks, valerian is an excellent sleep aid, and those who brave its bitter taste swear by it. A decoction is the form of preparation generally made with roots, however, a maceration (soaking in cold water instead of boiling) works better with valerian. To make the maceration, chop 1 ounce of fresh root into small pieces, pour 1 pint of cold water over the root, and let it soak for 8 to 10 hours. Strain it, and drink a cup an hour or two before bed. It also helps to relieve restlessness.

Other effective methods for taking valerian is in powdered form by capsule or as a tincture. A standard dose for valerian by capsule is 500 to 900 mg, however, try a smaller dose of half these amounts, first. If you are using a tincture, the standard dose is 1 to 2 teaspoons and like the capsule, take a

---

46. Susan Curtis and Louise Green, *Home Herbal: The Ultimate Guide to Cooking, Brewing, and Blending Your Own Herbs* (New York: Dorling Kindersley, 2011), 126.

smaller dose the first time you try it. Whether you are using a capsule or tincture, take it about two hours before bed. Valerian combines well with chamomile, lavender, or St. John's wort as a sleep aid.

VALERIAN BEDTIME TINCTURE

1 cup dried valerian root, chopped

¼ cup dried lavender flowers, crumbled

1 pint 80 to 100 proof alcohol

Chop the valerian root into small pieces. Place the herbs in a jar, pour in the alcohol to cover the plant material, close, and shake for 1 to 2 minutes. Set aside for 2 to 4 weeks, shaking the jar every other day. Strain out the herbs and store in dark glass bottles in a cool, dark place.

....

Valerian aids heart health by lowering blood pressure and increasing blood flow to the heart. Check with your doctor before using it for this purpose, especially if you are taking any medication for your heart or blood pressure.

The antispasmodic properties of valerian relieve menstrual and stomach cramps, abdominal pain, and nervous indigestion. It eases anxiety-produced hives, and in general, fortifies the nervous system. In addition, valerian can ease hiccups.

VALERIAN EASE THE TENSION TEA

1 teaspoon fresh valerian root, chopped

2 cups boiling water

1½ teaspoons fresh lemon balm leaves, chopped

Simmer the valerian root for 20 minutes. Place the lemon balm leaves in a jar and then pour in the water and valerian root. Steep for 20 minutes, strain, and drink when it is cool.

....

Drink two cups of tea a day or make a tincture and take one half to one teaspoon of it twice a day for a week. To help relieve nervous tension, make a cup of the tea and add ½ teaspoon of peppermint. The tea or a maceration are also helpful in providing relief from headaches, especially migraine.

How to Use the Essential Oils

The color of valerian essential oil ranges from olive to brown. It has a warm, woody, and balsamic scent. This oil can be used to ease strained muscles and relax muscle spasms. It also relieves the joint pain and inflammation of arthritis, rheumatism, and rheumatoid arthritis. See the profile on yarrow for a blend to ease pain. Alternatively, try the Bedtime/Relax Time Massage Oil to reduce swelling and inflammation associated with these conditions as well as for stress relief and general relaxation.

Bedtime/Relax Time Valerian Massage Oil

5 drops lavender essential oil

1 drop lemon balm essential oil

1 drop valerian essential oil

1 tablespoon carrier oil

Mix the essential oils together and then combine with the carrier oil.

....

A massage with valerian essential oil releases the tightness and discomfort in facial muscles that can occur with temporomandibular joint pain (TMJ). Because it is potent, use only 1 drop of valerian essential oil in 1 ounce of carrier oil for use on the face.

Valerian is instrumental for relieving the discomfort of sciatica either as a bath soak or as a warm compress. Mix 5 drops of valerian essential oil with 2 cups of coarse sea or Epsom salts. For a compress, mix 2 drops of essential oil in 1 quart of hot water. Give the mixture a good swish, dip in a washcloth, and then place it on the sore area.

Valerian Calming Bedtime Bath Blend

4 drops chamomile essential oil

3 drops clary essential oil

2 drops valerian essential oil

2 drops lavender essential oil

1 ounce carrier oil

Mix the essential oils together and then combine with the carrier oil.

....

Whether you need headache relief or just want to relax, the Valerian Headache Diffuser Blend is sure to reduce stress and promote a good night's sleep.

Valerian Headache Diffuser Blend

10 drops lavender essential oil

8 drops chamomile essential oil

1 drop valerian essential oil

Combine the oils and let the blend mature for about 1 week.

Yarrow

(Achillea millefolium L.)

Also known as: Blood Wort, Common Yarrow, Milfoil, Nosebleed, Thousand Leaf

To the Greeks, yarrow was an important medicinal herb that was named in honor of the hero Achilles who was said to have used it to heal the wounds of his fellow soldiers at Troy. Although the Romans also used it to stanch bleeding on the battlefield and called it *Herba Militaris*, they used yarrow more often for common things such as nosebleeds.[47] Whether or not it was used during the legendary battle of Troy, yarrow was a staple in battlefield medical kits from the time of the Crusades up through the Civil War.

Yarrow has also been known for its variety of other medicinal uses. Both the ancient Greeks and Renaissance Britons sung its praises for healing and it came to be known as Cure-All.[48] It was extolled for the treatment of rheumatism. In America, the Shakers used yarrow in a range of remedies that they sold through their herb business. This plant has been a powerhouse for creating a range of dyes including golds, grays, greens, yellows, and black.

Medicinal Uses

Acne, amenorrhea, boils, bruises, colds, cuts and scrapes, digestive system support, eczema, fever, flu, hair care, hemorrhoids, indigestion, infection, inflammation, insect repellent, menorrhagia, menstrual cramps, menstrual cycle problems, nosebleed, rheumatism, rheumatoid arthritis, scars, skin care, sore throat, sprains, stomachache or pain, varicose veins

Precautions and Contraindications

The herb: Avoid during pregnancy and while breastfeeding; may cause allergic reaction in those sensitive to ragweed and related plants; large doses may induce headache; use in moderation; do not use when taking medications that slow blood clotting.

The essential oils: Herbal precautions also apply.

Parts of Plant Used

Herbal remedies: Leaves and flowers

Essential oils: Entire plant

Culinary purposes: Leaves

---

47. John Andrew Eastman, *The Book of Field and Roadside: Open-country Weeds, Trees, and Wildflowers of Eastern North America* (Mechanicsburg, PA: Stackpole Books, 2003), 320.
48. Gladstar, *Medicinal Herbs*, 214.

Growing and Harvesting

Yarrow is a slender, upright plant that grows one to three feet tall with a branching, smooth, green stem. Its pinnate leaves are ferny and covered with soft hairs. Its small white to pinkish flowers grow in wide umbel clusters and bloom from midsummer to autumn. The plant has a pleasant, sweet smell.

Type	Zone	Light	Soil	Moisture	Height	Spacing
Perennial	2	Full sun to partial shade	Any	Moist	1–3'	18"

Yarrow prefers full sun but will grow in partial shade. Easily grown from seed, yarrow is happy in almost any soil and does well in containers. It readily self-seeds but can also be propagated by root division. Yarrow increases essential oil production in other plants growing nearby, making it especially good for aromatic herbs. It attracts a range of good bugs including ladybugs, hoverflies, and predatory wasps. Yarrow's blooming period can be extended by removing flowers before they set seed. Stems with leaves and flowers can be hung to dry. Yarrow is good for the compost pile because it helps to speed decomposition.

How to Use the Herb

As history attests, yarrow heals wounds. In addition to coagulating the blood, it has anti-inflammatory and antiseptic properties that keep wounds from getting infected. However, always be sure to clean the cut first. A yarrow tincture works just as well as iodine and it helps to relieve any associated pain. A poultice of fresh leaves will stanch the bleeding of a wound or a nosebleed. Also, dried flowers and leaves can be ground together to make a first-aid powder that can be sprinkled on an open wound. A little powder inside the nostril can slow a nosebleed.

Combining yarrow with peppermint in tea is an effective treatment to relieve cold and flu symptoms. This tea also helps soothe a sore throat. Additionally, yarrow stimulates blood flow to the surface of the skin promoting sweating and reducing fever. For a fever, drink half a cup every thirty minutes to bring on a sweat.

FEVER REDUCING YARROW TEA

1 teaspoon dried yarrow flowers and leaves, crumbled

1 teaspoon dried peppermint leaves, crumbled

1 cup boiling water

Combine the herbs and pour the water over them. Steep for 10 to 20 minutes and strain. Even though peppermint reduces the bitterness of yarrow, a little honey also helps.

Odd as it may seem, while yarrow can reduce heavy menstrual bleeding it can also stimulate a late period and help with amenorrhea. In addition, its antispasmodic properties relieve menstrual cramps.

Yarrow Menstrual Aid Tea

1½ teaspoons dried yarrow flowers and leaves, crumbled

½ teaspoon dried lemon balm leaves, crumbled

1 cup boiling water

Combine the herbs and pour the water over them. Steep 10 to 15 minutes and strain. Add honey to taste. When making this tea for amenorrhea, use sage instead of lemon balm.

Yarrow's antiseptic and anti-inflammatory properties are also helpful for treating bruises and sprains. Apply a poultice of leaves to a sprain to stop the swelling. Alternatively, a cloth moistened with a yarrow tincture can be applied.

A yarrow poultice is also good for drawing pus out of boils or infected cuts. Another method for this is to use a yarrow infusion as a soak if the boil or cut is on a part of the body (hand, arm, foot) that is easily immersed in a pan of water. The infusion should be as warm as possible but not so hot that it burns or is uncomfortable.

The astringent qualities of this plant make it an effective salve for treating hemorrhoids. Apply it several times a day. Instead of a salve, an infusion can be used in a sitz bath. The salve can treat bruises, too. A yarrow liniment helps to ease varicose veins. Compresses made with a yarrow infusion used on the legs especially during pregnancy reduces swelling and discomfort.

Although yarrow does not have a wide culinary use, pick a few young leaves to add to a green salad. The bitters in yarrow leaves make it a tonic for the digestive system. It fights inflammation and infections of the stomach lining and the intestines. Yarrow's antispasmodic properties relieve stomachaches. To avoid the bitter taste of yarrow, brew the tea with other herbs, such as peppermint as in the Fever-Reducing Yarrow Tea or try the following infusion.

Soothe the Belly Yarrow Infusion

3 tablespoons dried yarrow flowers, crumbled

2 tablespoons dried chamomile flowers, crumbled

1 tablespoon dried angelica root, chopped

1 quart water

Place the angelica root in the water and simmer for 15 to 20 minutes. Place the yarrow and chamomile in a large jar or pitcher and carefully pour in the water and angelica root. Let it steep for 30 to 60 minutes, and then strain.

As an alternative to the tea, make a yarrow tincture. For indigestion take one quarter to a half teaspoon of it three times a day. For help with digestive system infections, make an infusion with equal parts yarrow and peppermint. Drink two cups a day. Yarrow also helps remove toxins from the body and purify the blood.

The astringent properties of this herb make it good for skin care. Yarrow tea can be used as a facial rinse that soothes the inflammation of acne. Combine it with chamomile for a facial steam that is effective for unclogging and cleaning the pores. A yarrow infusion makes a good cleanser for oily skin and a conditioner for oily hair. While gardening or doing anything outside, an insect repellent is always helpful. Before going outside, spray Yarrow Insect Repellent Infusion on exposed skin and rub it in.

YARROW INSECT REPELLENT INFUSION

¼ cup yarrow dried flowers, crumbled

¼ cup lavender dried leaves, crumbled

2 cups boiling water

Combine the herbs and pour in water. Steep for 30 to 60 minutes and then strain into a spray bottle.

How to Use the Essential Oils

Yarrow essential oil has a sweet, herbaceous scent. Its color ranges from dark blue to greenish.

Like a yarrow infusion, the essential oil works well for skin care, especially acne and eczema. Apricot kernel and jojoba carrier oils are good choices for this application. This mix can also help reduce scars.

Yarrow blends well with Roman chamomile and valerian to create a massage oil for rheumatism, rheumatoid arthritis, and varicose veins, which will also help circulation in general.

EASE THE PAIN YARROW MASSAGE OIL

3 drops yarrow essential oil

2 drops Roman chamomile essential oil

2 drops valerian essential oil

1 tablespoon carrier oil

Mix the essential oils together and then combine with the carrier oil.

CONCLUSION

While still considered an alternative medicine, we have seen that for thousands of years herbal remedies were the only medicine available. The use of herbal remedies has weathered an up-and-down relationship with the medical establishment as well as the devastation of witch hunts. Herbs and essential oils may have taken a back seat to chemicals in the manufacture of many drugs but that, too, is changing as more people seek a natural approach to healing.

That natural approach extends to our gardens. Chemicals used on our plants or in the soil ultimately end up inside of us. Composting and going organic may require a little more work, and it does not produce uniform, picture-perfect plants. However, by going organic we are guaranteeing that we will have the best possible herbs to put in our food and our remedies without causing harm to the environment. Also, while gardens take work, it is work that puts us outdoors in the fresh air and it provides good exercise.

Whether it is an outdoor garden or containers on a porch or windowsill, tending to plants makes us more aware of nature's cycles, which is healing and brings balance to our lives. Gardening provides the perfect opportunity to slow down and be in the moment. Watching the herbs we nurture grow and mature, and harvesting what we have grown fosters a meaningful satisfaction. While gardening connects us with the natural world, it also puts us in touch with ourselves on a fundamental soul level.

Gardening teaches us patience. It takes time to grow things. Also, we may not have success with every plant we want to grow. Rosemary is one that still eludes me, but someday I will have a healthy plant that I can shepherd through the winter.

Just as cooking a special meal for those we love is satisfying and rewarding, so too is working with herbs and making remedies for ourselves and our families. Gardening and working with herbs takes us outside of ourselves. It harkens back to the wise folk who cared for their village neighbors, and it creates a connection through time that binds us to the earth and to each other. I find it amazing that something as simple as an herb can be so powerful in so many ways.

Herbs for Ailments, Conditions, and Support for Good Health

Abdominal Pain

basil

valerian

Acne

borage

caraway

chamomile

clary

lavender

lemon balm

lemongrass

peppermint

rosemary

sage

spearmint

thyme

yarrow

Amenorrhea

angelica

clary

dill

fennel

parsley

sage

yarrow

Anemia

parsley

Anorexia

angelica

coriander

Anxiety

angelica

basil

coriander

hyssop

lavender

lemon balm

marjoram

spearmint

St. John's wort

valerian

Appetite Stimulant

angelica
anise
bay
caraway
coriander
fennel
marjoram
parsley
spearmint
thyme

Arthritis

angelica
bay
cayenne
chamomile
coriander
lemongrass
marjoram
parsley
rosemary
sage
St. John's wort
thyme
valerian

Asthma

anise
basil
bay
clary
hyssop
lemon balm
marjoram
peppermint

rosemary
sage
thyme

Athlete's Foot

bay
garlic
lavender
lemongrass
rosemary
thyme

Bad Breath

anise
basil
caraway
coriander
dill
parsley
peppermint
rosemary
sage
spearmint
thyme

Belching

caraway
chamomile
fennel
peppermint
spearmint

Bladder Infection / Inflammation

borage
parsley

Bloating

anise
bay
caraway
cayenne
chamomile
coriander
fennel
hyssop
lavender
thyme

Blood Pressure

garlic
lemon balm
valerian

Blood Sugar

garlic

Boils

borage
caraway
clary
lavender
sage
thyme
yarrow

Breast Problems

chamomile
dill

Breastfeeding Problems

anise
caraway

dill
fennel

Breastfeeding Weaning

parsley
sage

Bronchitis

angelica
anise
basil
bay
borage
caraway
dill
garlic
hyssop
lavender
lemon balm
marjoram
peppermint
rosemary

Bruises

bay
caraway
fennel
hyssop
lavender
marjoram
parsley
St. John's wort
yarrow

Burns

chamomile
lavender

peppermint
rosemary
spearmint
St. John's wort

Cardiovascular System Support
angelica
cayenne
coriander
garlic
rosemary
valerian

Carpal Tunnel
bay
cayenne
marjoram
sage

Catarrh
borage
caraway
hyssop
marjoram

Cellulite
fennel

Chest Congestion
angelica
anise
borage
cayenne
dill
hyssop
lavender
lemon balm
marjoram

peppermint
rosemary
spearmint
thyme

Chicken Pox
St. John's wort

Chilblains
cayenne
marjoram
peppermint

Childbirth
St. John's wort

Chills
cayenne

Cholesterol
cayenne
garlic

Chronic Fatigue
basil
borage
lavender
marjoram

Cold Sores
hyssop
lavender
St. John's wort

Colds
angelica
anise
basil

bay
borage
cayenne
dill
garlic
hyssop
lavender
lemon balm
marjoram
peppermint
rosemary
sage
spearmint
thyme
yarrow

Colic
chamomile
dill

Colitis
chamomile

Constipation
fennel
marjoram

Cough
angelica
anise
basil
borage
caraway
clary
dill
fennel
garlic

hyssop
lemon balm
marjoram
peppermint
sage
spearmint
thyme

Crohn's Disease
chamomile

Cuts and Scrapes
cayenne
chamomile
hyssop
lavender
rosemary
sage
St. John's wort
thyme
yarrow

Dandruff
bay
chamomile
clary
parsley
rosemary
sage

Dermatitis
borage
hyssop
lavender
lemon balm
peppermint
St. John's wort

Diarrhea
peppermint
sage

Digestive System Support
basil
bay
caraway
cayenne
chamomile
coriander
dill
garlic
hyssop
lemon balm
lemongrass
marjoram
parsley
peppermint
sage
spearmint
thyme
yarrow

Ear Infection
garlic

Earache
basil
chamomile
thyme

Eczema
borage
chamomile
clary
hyssop

lavender
lemon balm
rosemary
sage
St. John's wort
thyme
yarrow

Edema
fennel

Expectorants
angelica
anise
borage
fennel
hyssop
peppermint
thyme

Eye Problems
chamomile
fennel
parsley

Fainting
basil
rosemary

Fever
borage
chamomile
coriander
hyssop
lemon balm
lemongrass
yarrow

Fibromyalgia

cayenne

Flatulence

angelica

anise

basil

bay

caraway

cayenne

clary

coriander

dill

fennel

hyssop

lavender

lemongrass

marjoram

parsley

peppermint

rosemary

sage

spearmint

thyme

Flu

basil

bay

cayenne

garlic

hyssop

lavender

lemon balm

marjoram

peppermint

rosemary

sage

thyme

yarrow

Gallstones

peppermint

spearmint

Gastritis

angelica

chamomile

coriander

Gastroenteritis

lemongrass

Gingivitis

basil

peppermint

sage

spearmint

thyme

Gout

coriander

fennel

parsley

peppermint

Hair Care

basil

bay

chamomile

clary

parsley

rosemary

St. John's wort

yarrow

Hangover

cayenne

thyme

Hay Fever

basil

chamomile

marjoram

parsley

thyme

Head Lice

anise

lavender

lemongrass

Headache

angelica

basil

cayenne

chamomile

clary

coriander

dill

lavender

lemon balm

lemongrass

marjoram

peppermint

rosemary

sage

thyme

valerian

Heartburn

angelica

chamomile

coriander

dill

fennel

marjoram

peppermint

spearmint

Hemorrhoids

lavender

yarrow

Herpes

hyssop

lavender

lemon balm

St. John's wort

Hiccups

dill

valerian

Hives

valerian

Hyperactivity

spearmint

Immune System Support

cayenne

garlic

lemon balm

rosemary

thyme

Indigestion

angelica

anise

basil
bay
caraway
chamomile
clary
coriander
dill
fennel
hyssop
lavender
lemon balm
lemongrass
marjoram
parsley
peppermint
rosemary
sage
spearmint
thyme
valerian
yarrow

Infection

basil
coriander
garlic
hyssop
lemon balm
peppermint
rosemary
St. John's wort
thyme
yarrow

Inflammation

chamomile
hyssop
lavender

lemon balm
parsley
peppermint
rosemary
sage
St. John's wort
thyme
valerian
yarrow

Insect Bites and Stings

basil
bay
chamomile
garlic
lavender
lemon balm
lemongrass
parsley
peppermint
sage
St. John's wort

Insect Repellent

basil
bay
hyssop
lemongrass
peppermint
yarrow

Insomnia

basil
chamomile
lavender
lemon balm
marjoram
valerian

Irritable Bowel Syndrome (IBS)
angelica
caraway
peppermint

Jock Itch
bay
garlic
lavender
lemongrass

Joint Stiffness
bay
cayenne
coriander
lavender
marjoram

Kidney Stones
fennel
parsley

Laryngitis
caraway
clary
lavender
lemongrass
sage

Lymph Circulation
coriander
fennel
rosemary

Mastitis
chamomile
parsley

Menopausal Discomforts
anise
borage
clary
fennel
sage
St. John's wort
thyme

Menorrhagia
yarrow

Menstrual Cramps
angelica
anise
caraway
clary
dill
lavender
lemon balm
marjoram
parsley
sage
thyme
valerian
yarrow

Menstrual Cycle Problems
angelica
anise
fennel
marjoram
parsley
yarrow

Mental Fatigue
lemongrass
rosemary

Migraine

cayenne

clary

lavender

lemon balm

marjoram

rosemary

thyme

valerian

Motion Sickness

basil

marjoram

peppermint

spearmint

Mouth Ulcers

basil

rosemary

sage

Muscle Ache or Pain

basil

bay

cayenne

chamomile

clary

coriander

lavender

lemongrass

marjoram

peppermint

rosemary

sage

spearmint

thyme

valerian

Muscle Strain

lavender

marjoram

peppermint

rosemary

St. John's wort

valerian

Nail Fungus

lavender

Nasal Congestion

anise

basil

bay

cayenne

fennel

hyssop

marjoram

peppermint

rosemary

spearmint

thyme

Nausea

basil

caraway

chamomile

coriander

fennel

marjoram

peppermint

spearmint

Nerve Pain

cayenne

coriander

lavender

lemongrass
peppermint
spearmint

Nervous Exhaustion

lemongrass
rosemary

Nervous System Support

basil
coriander
hyssop
lemon balm
marjoram
peppermint
rosemary
spearmint
St. John's wort
valerian

Nervous Tension

angelica
chamomile
clary
dill
hyssop
lavender
St. John's wort
valerian

Nosebleed

yarrow

Postnatal Depression

anise
caraway
dill
fennel

Premenstrual Syndrome (PMS)

borage
clary
fennel
lemon balm
marjoram
parsley
St. John's wort
thyme

Psoriasis

angelica
borage
clary
lavender
lemon balm
rosemary
sage
St. John's wort
thyme

Pyorrhea

fennel

Rashes

bay
borage
chamomile
peppermint

Raynaud's Disease

borage

Restlessness

lemon balm
valerian

Rheumatism

angelica
bay
chamomile
coriander
lavender
lemongrass
marjoram
parsley
rosemary
sage
St. John's wort
valerian
yarrow

Rheumatoid Arthritis

borage
cayenne
chamomile
valerian
yarrow

Ringworm

garlic
lavender
lemongrass

Scabies

anise
bay
caraway
lavender
lemongrass
peppermint
spearmint
St. John's wort
thyme

Scars

lavender
St. John's wort
yarrow

Sciatica

bay
lavender
marjoram
parsley
St. John's wort
thyme
valerian

Seasonal Affective Disorder (SAD)

lemon balm
St. John's wort

Shingles

cayenne
lemon balm
St. John's wort

Sinusitis

basil
garlic
lavender
marjoram
rosemary
thyme

Skin Care

angelica
bay
borage
caraway
chamomile

clary
coriander
fennel
hyssop
lavender
lemon balm
lemongrass
peppermint
sage
spearmint
St. John's wort
thyme
yarrow

Sleep Aid
anise
chamomile
dill
lavender
lemon balm
peppermint
spearmint
St. John's wort
valerian

Sore Throat
bay
cayenne
chamomile
clary
fennel
garlic
hyssop
lavender
lemongrass
marjoram
peppermint

rosemary
sage
spearmint
thyme
yarrow

Sprains
bay
chamomile
lavender
lemongrass
marjoram
peppermint
rosemary
St. John's wort
yarrow

Staph Infection
garlic

Sties
garlic
thyme

Stomach Ulcer
angelica
coriander
peppermint

Stomachache or Pain
angelica
anise
basil
caraway
chamomile
clary
coriander

fennel

lemon balm

lemongrass

peppermint

rosemary

sage

thyme

valerian

yarrow

Strep Throat

garlic

lavender

Stress

angelica

anise

basil

borage

chamomile

clary

coriander

hyssop

lavender

lemon balm

lemongrass

rosemary

St. John's wort

valerian

Stretch Marks

borage

Sunburn

chamomile

lavender

peppermint

St. John's wort

Teething Pain

chamomile

Temporomandibular Joint Pain (TMJ)

borage

coriander

marjoram

rosemary

valerian

Tonsillitis

clary

garlic

hyssop

lavender

peppermint

sage

thyme

Tooth Decay

bay

peppermint

spearmint

Toothache

chamomile

Upset Stomach

anise

caraway

chamomile

coriander

marjoram

peppermint

spearmint

Vaginitis / Vaginal Yeast Infection

bay
garlic
lavender
lemongrass
sage

Varicose Veins

rosemary
St. John's wort
yarrow

Warts

basil
garlic

Water Retention

angelica
fennel

APPENDIX B

Measurement Equivalents

The following tables will help you find the easiest way to measure ingredients. Please note in the Measurement Equivalents table that 16 ounces equals a pound in weight and a pint in volume.

Measurement Equivalents
1 tablespoon = 3 teaspoons
1/16 cup = 1 tablespoon
1/8 cup = 2 tablespoons
1/6 cup = 2 tablespoons + 2 teaspoons
1/4 cup = 4 tablespoons
1/3 cup = 5 tablespoons + 1 teaspoon
3/8 cup = 6 tablespoons
1/2 cup = 8 tablespoons
2/3 cup = 10 tablespoons + 2 teaspoons
3/4 cup = 12 tablespoons
1 cup = 16 tablespoons or 48 teaspoons
1 ounce = 2 tablespoons
4 ounces = 1/2 cup
8 ounces = 1 cup
1 pint = 2 cups or 16 ounces
1 quart = 2 pints or 4 cups or 32 ounces
1 gallon = 4 quarts
1 pound = 16 ounces
1/2 pound = 8 ounces
1/4 pound = 4 ounces

Essential Oil Measurement Conversion Chart			
20–24 drops	= 1 ml	= ¼ teaspoon	
40–48 drops	= 2 ml	= ½ teaspoon	
100 drops	= 5 ml	= 1 teaspoon	= ⅙ oz
200 drops	= 10 ml	= 2 teaspoons	= ⅓ oz
300 drops	= 15 ml	= 1 tablespoon	= ½ oz
600 drops	= 30 ml	= 2 tablespoons	= 1 ounce

Carrier to Essential Oil Dilution Ratios					
Carrier Oil	*5ml*	*10ml*	*15ml*	*30ml*	*Ratio*
Essential Oil	1–2 drops	2–3 drops	3–5 drops	6–10 drops	1%
Essential Oil	2–3 drops	4–7 drops	6–10 drops	12–20 drops	2%
Essential Oil	3–5 drops	6–10 drops	9–16 drops	18–32 drops	3%
Essential Oil	4–7 drops	8–14 drops	12–20 drops	24–40 drops	4%

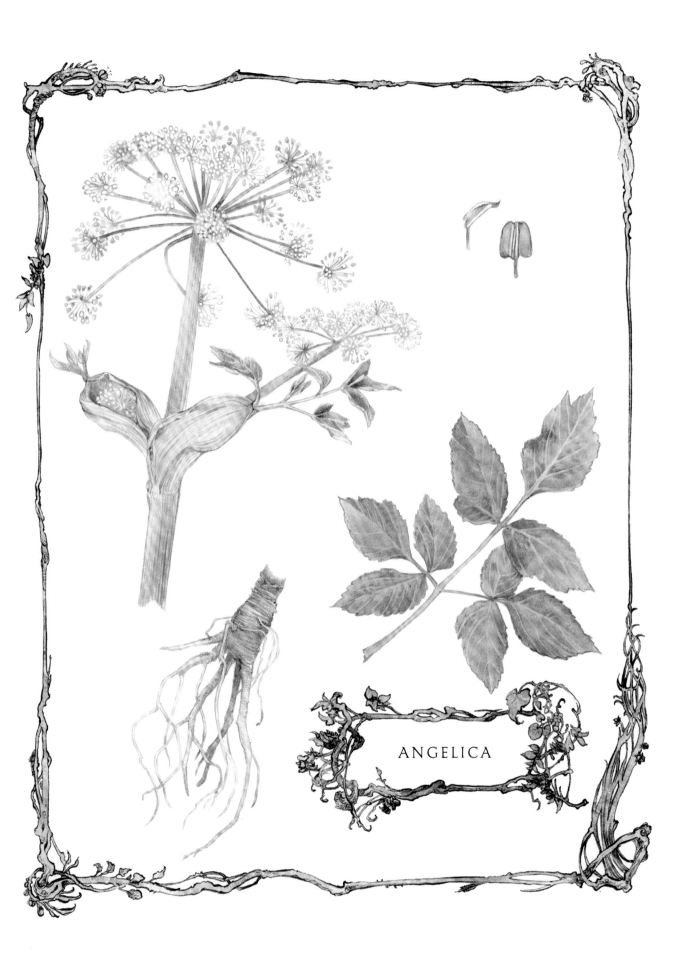

ANGELICA

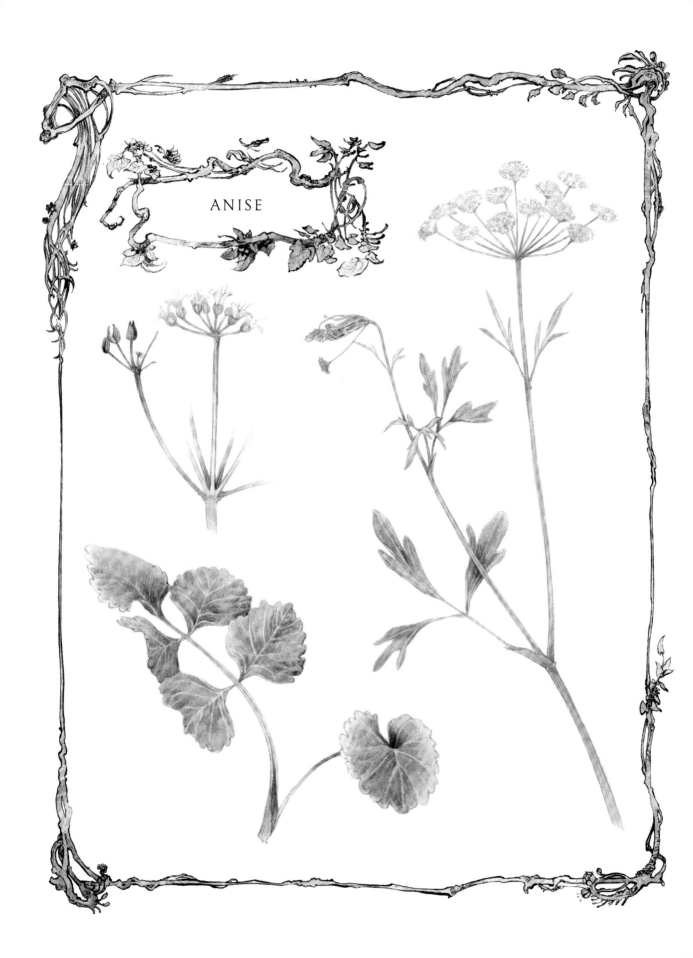

ANISE

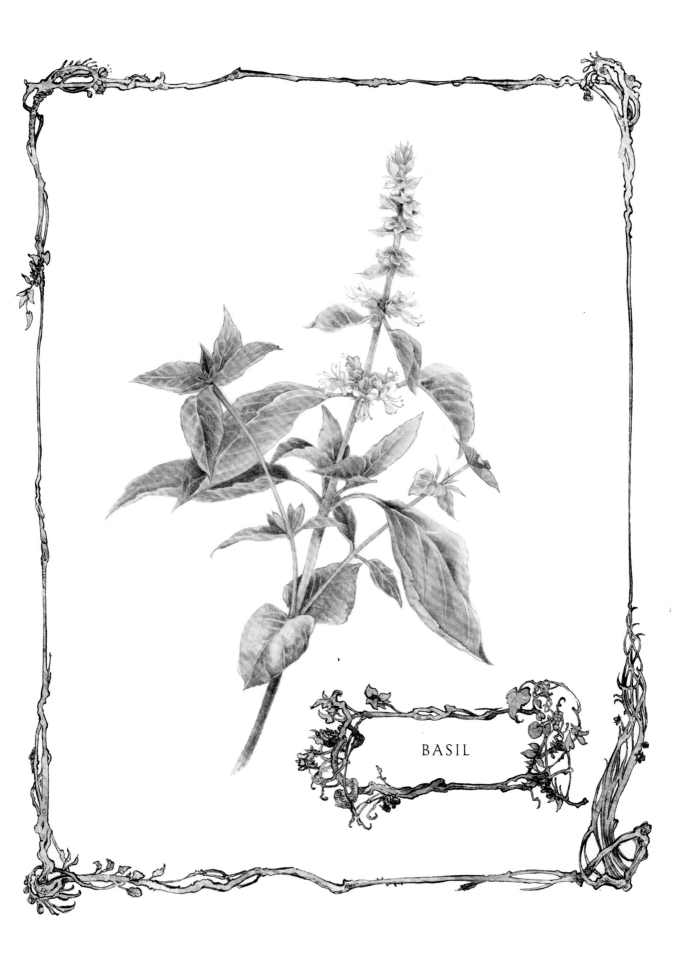

BASIL

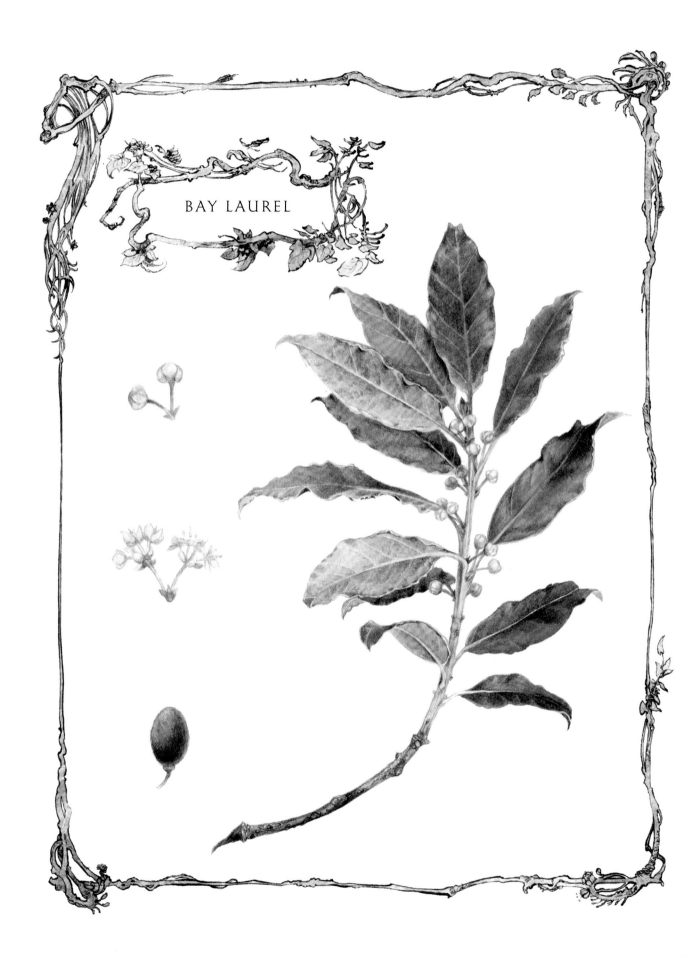

BAY LAUREL

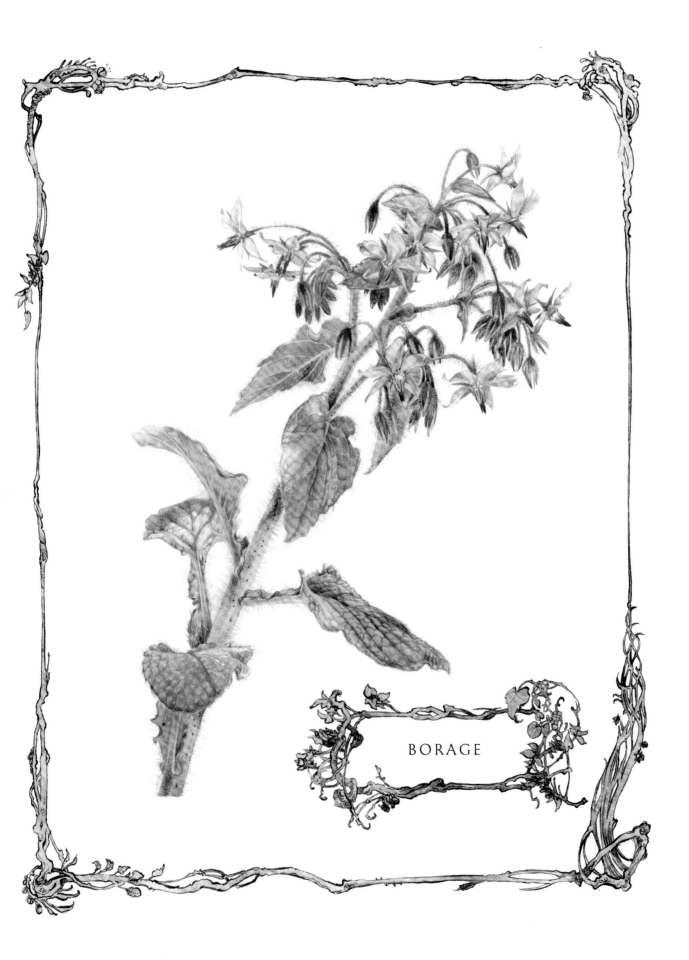

BORAGE

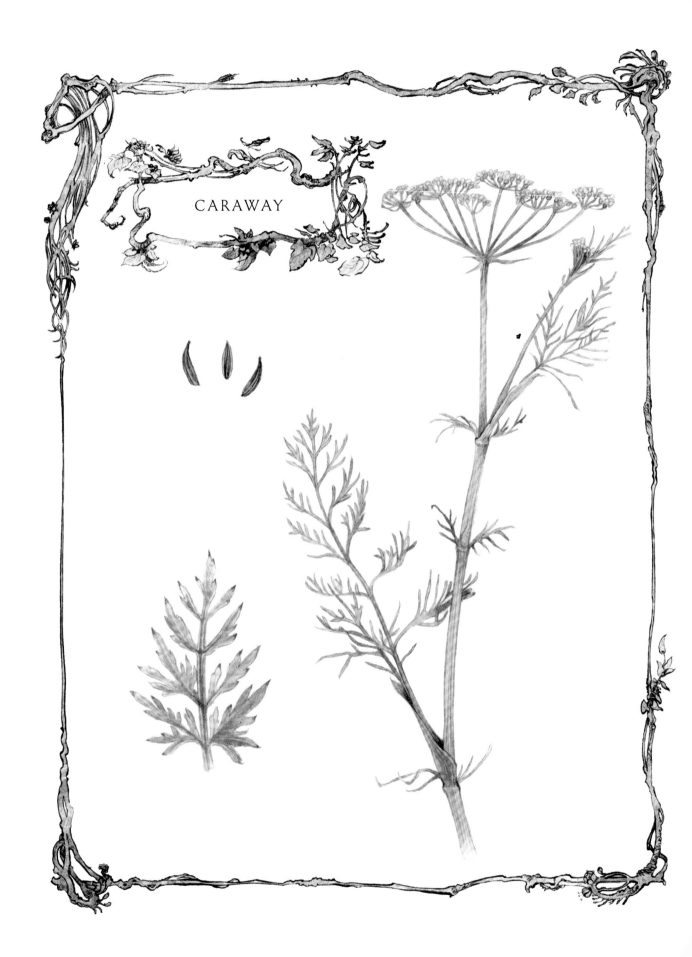

CARAWAY

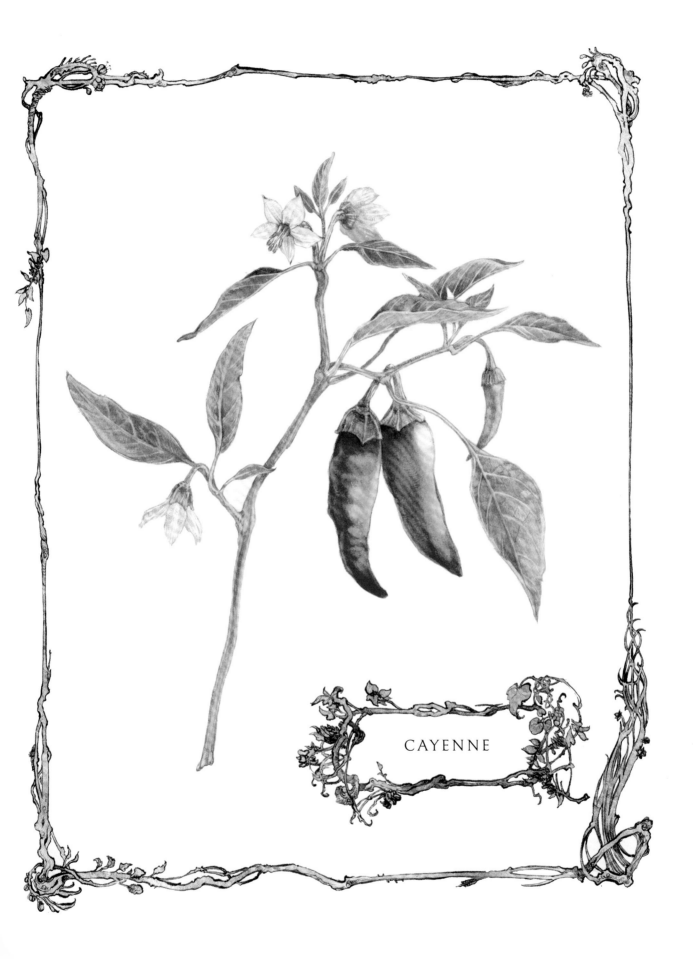

CAYENNE

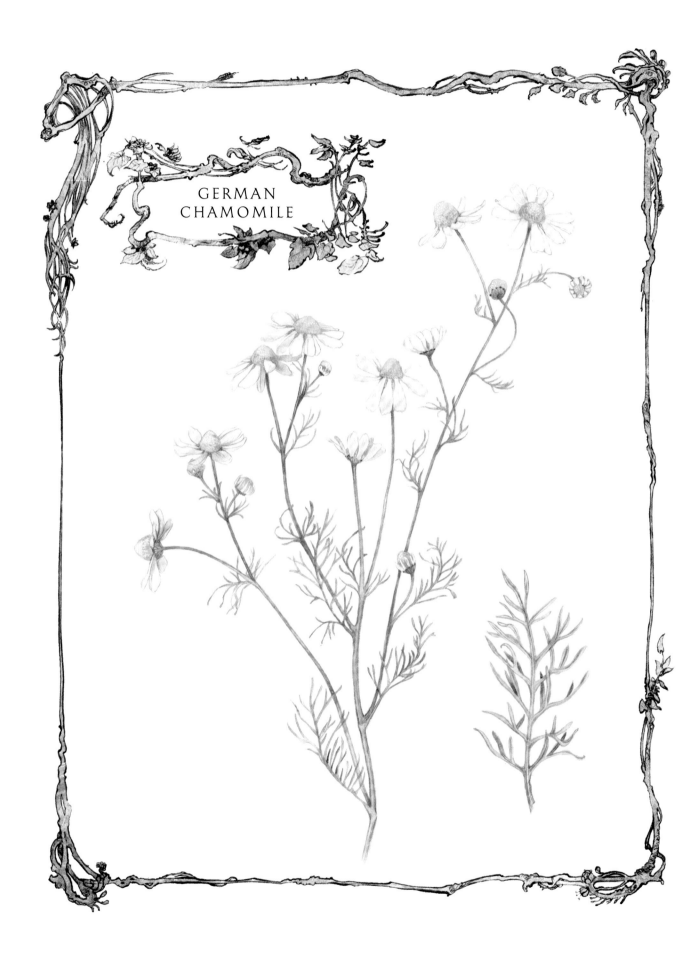

GERMAN
CHAMOMILE

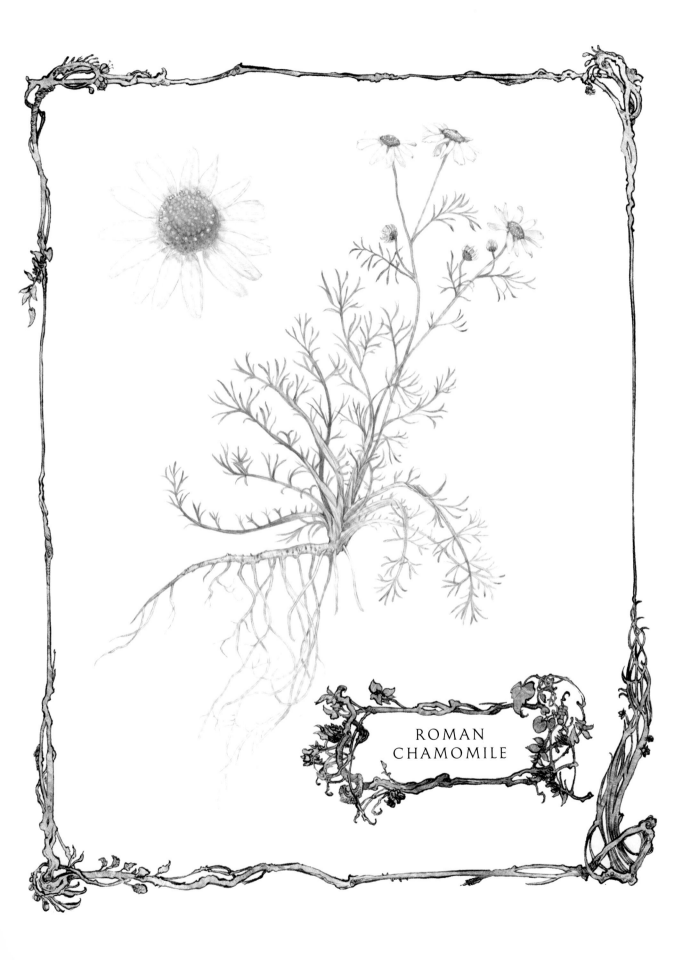

ROMAN
CHAMOMILE

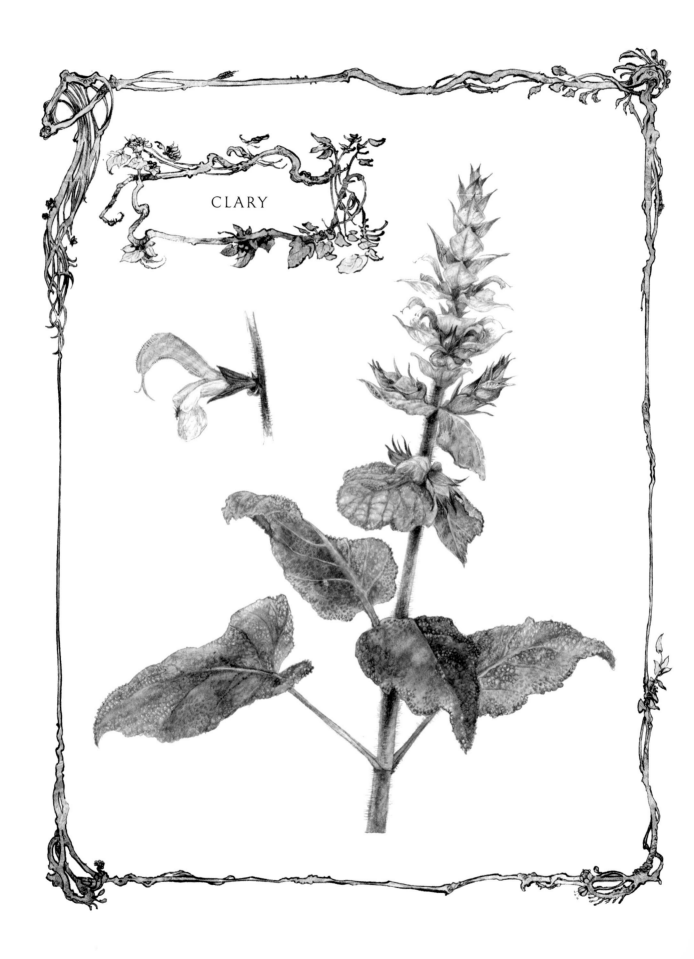

CLARY

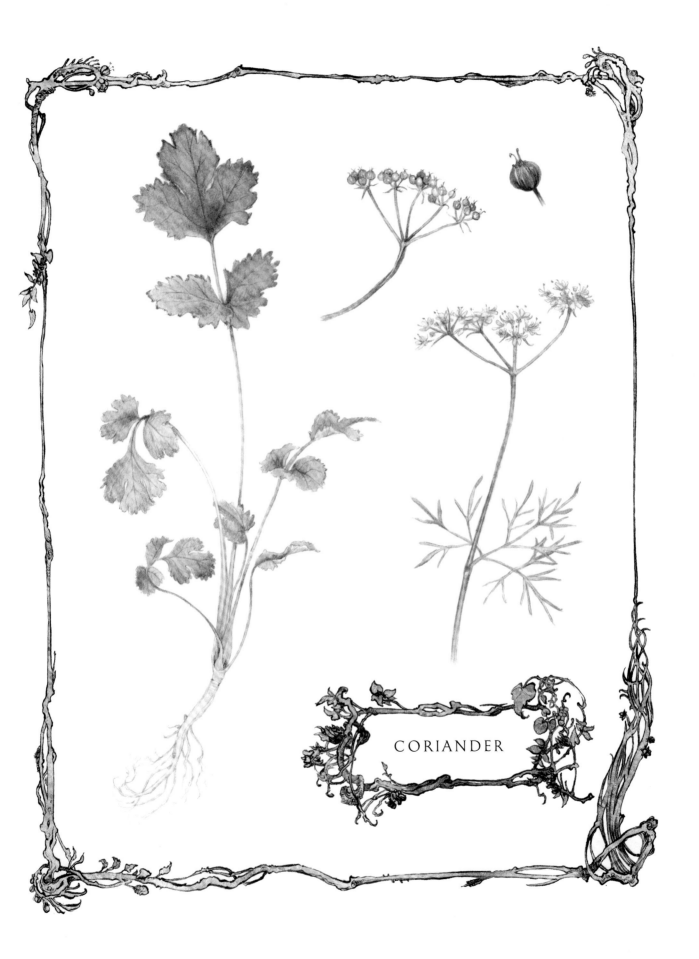

CORIANDER

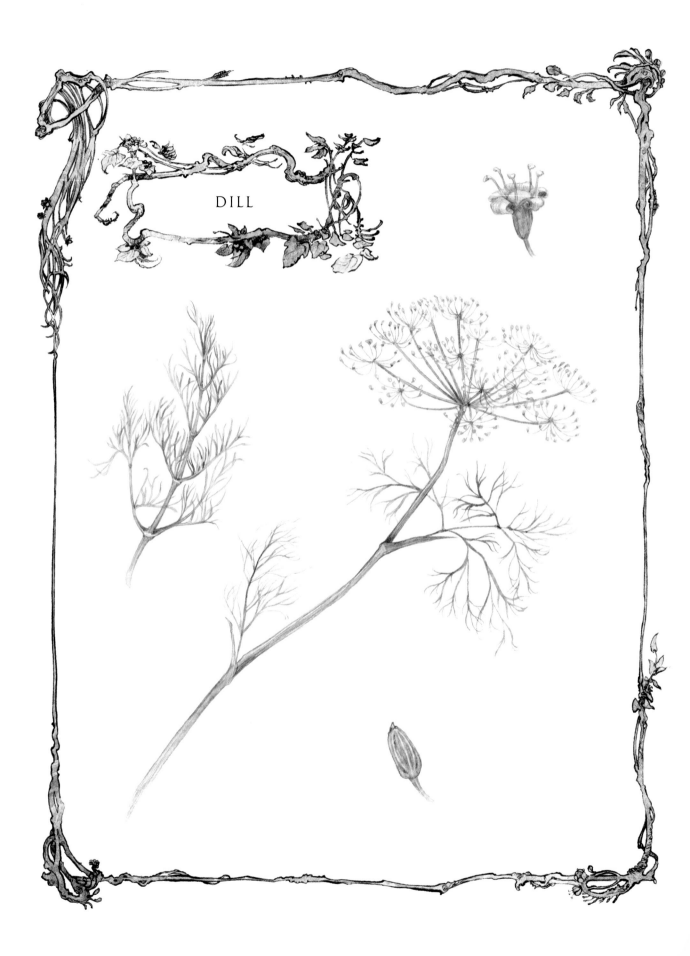

DILL

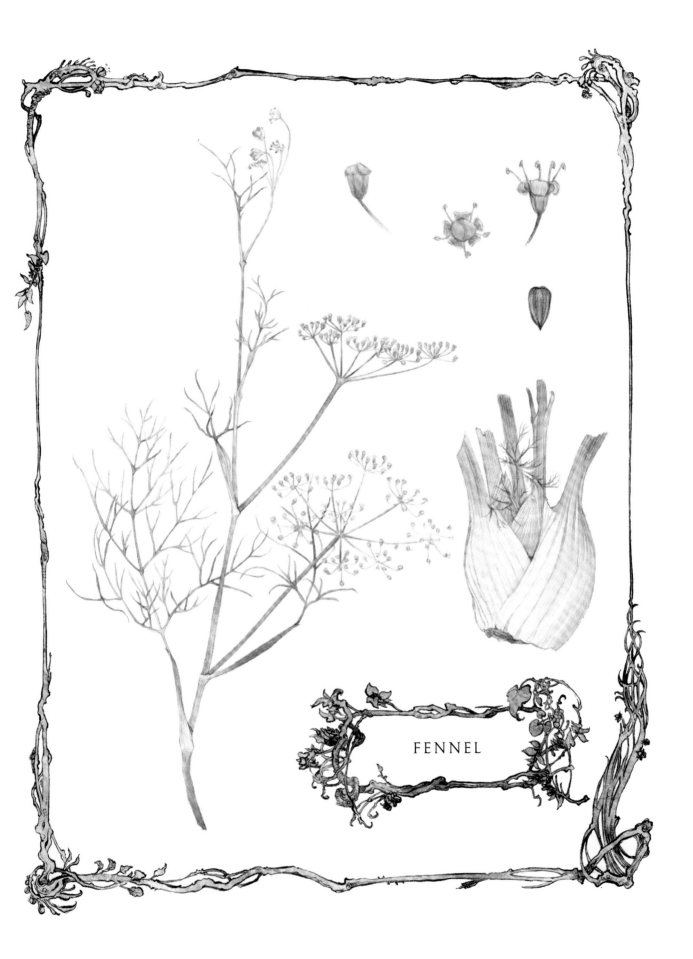

FENNEL

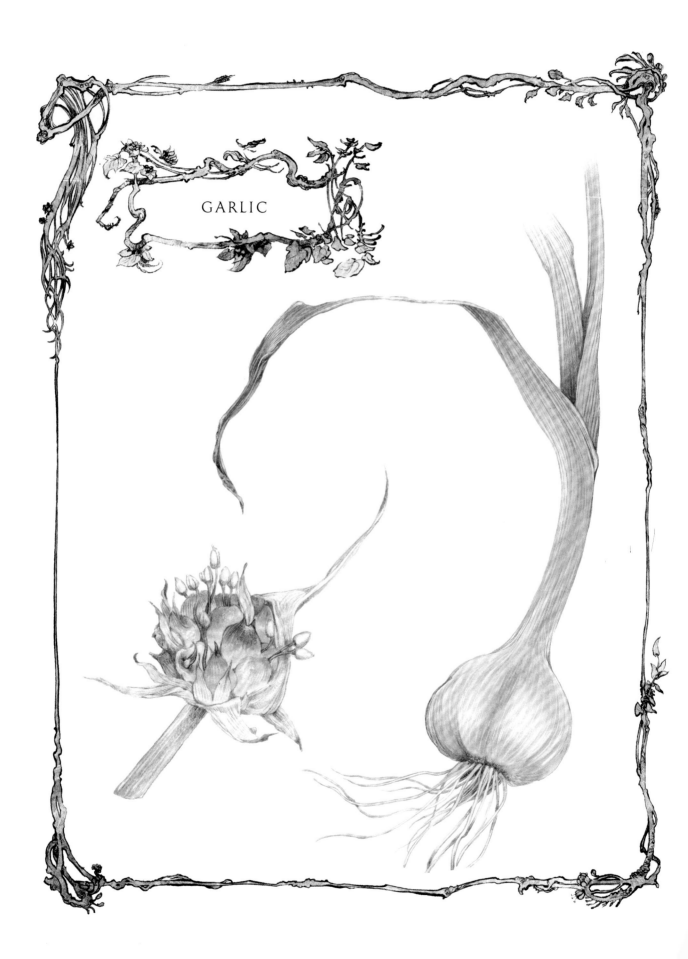

GARLIC

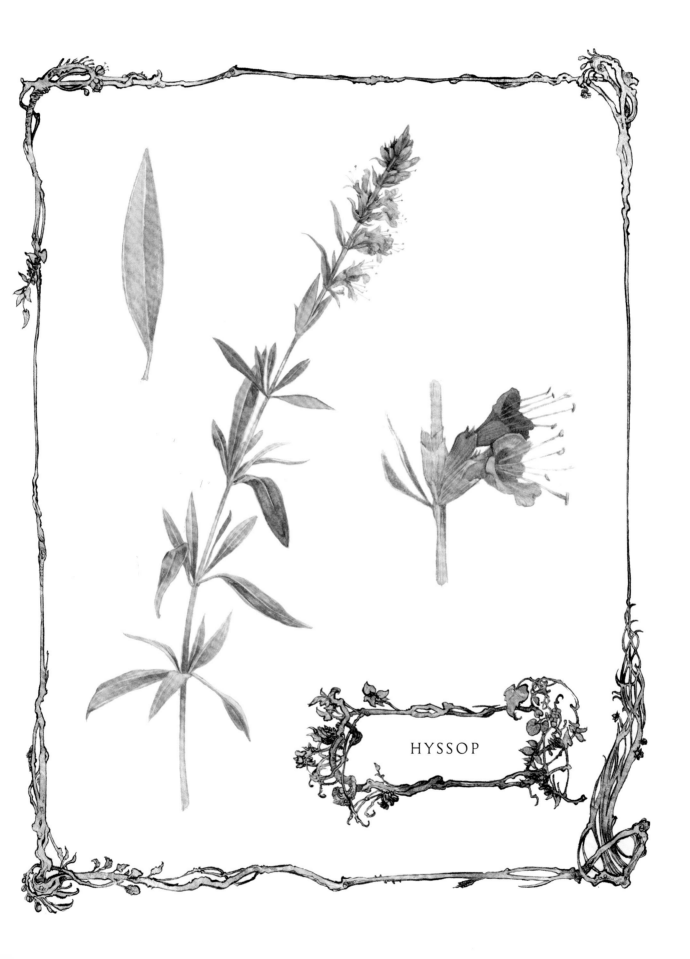

HYSSOP

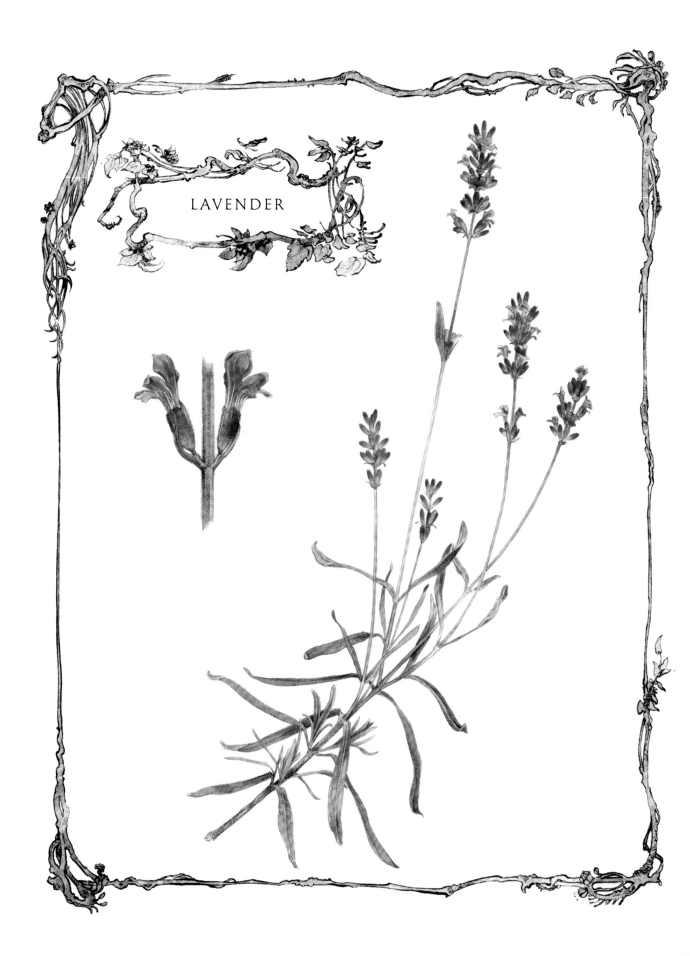

LAVENDER

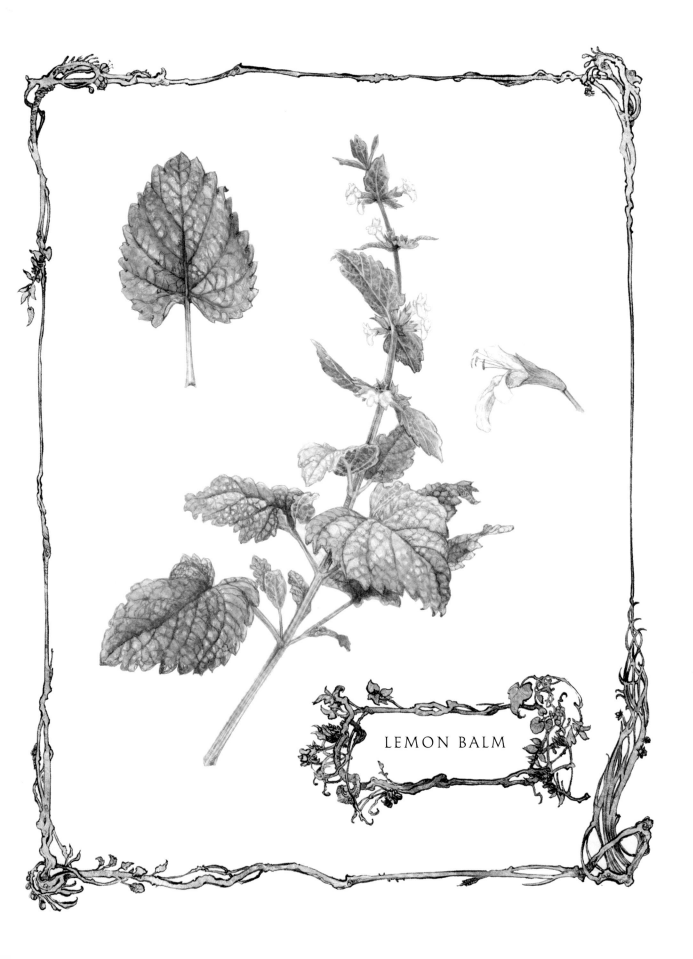

LEMON BALM

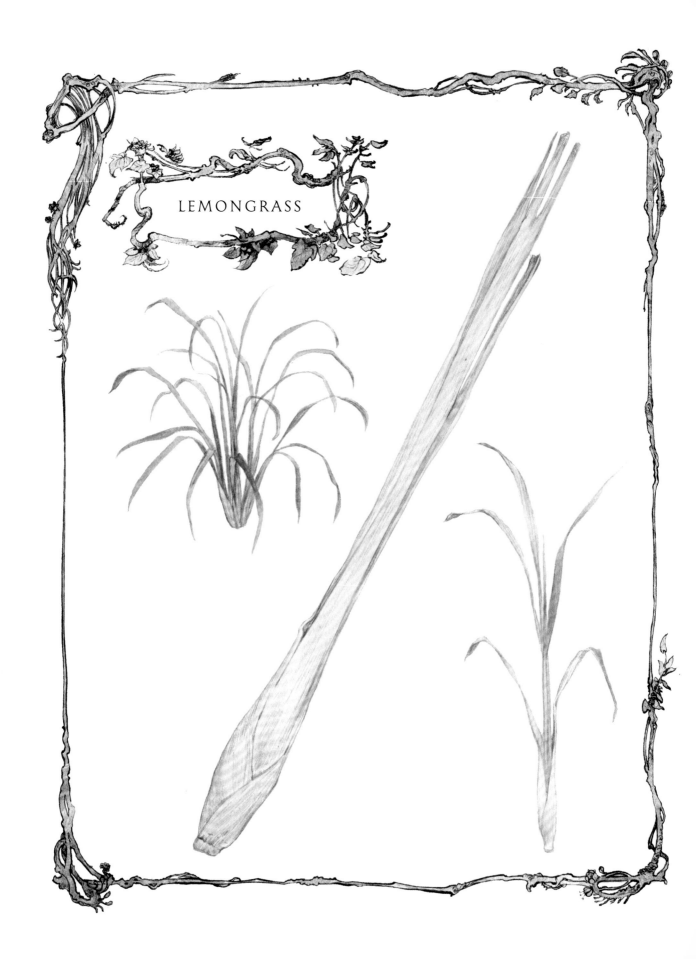

LEMONGRASS

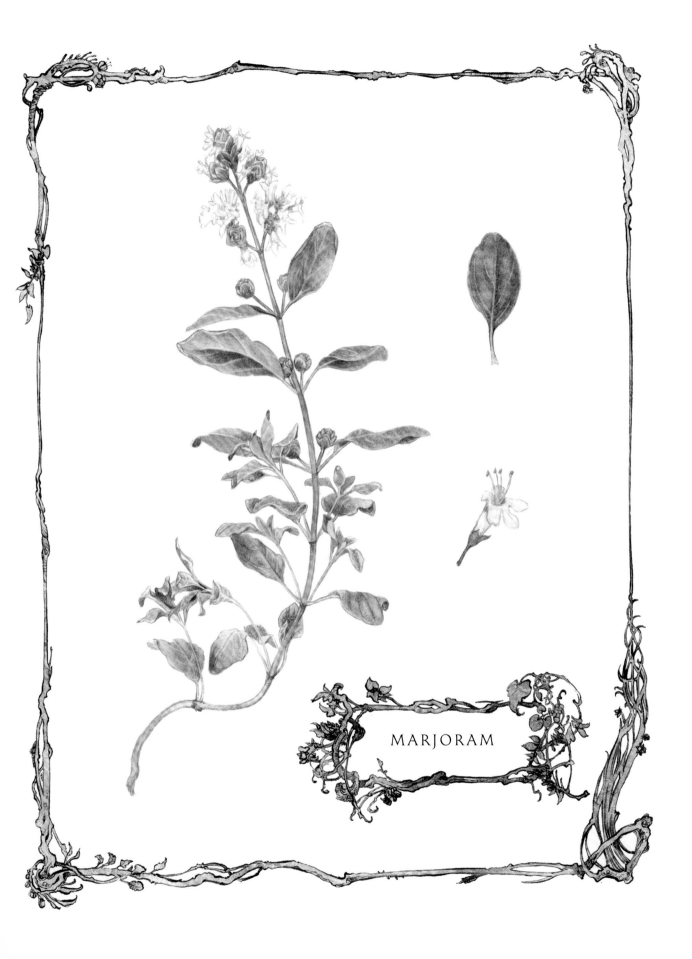

MARJORAM

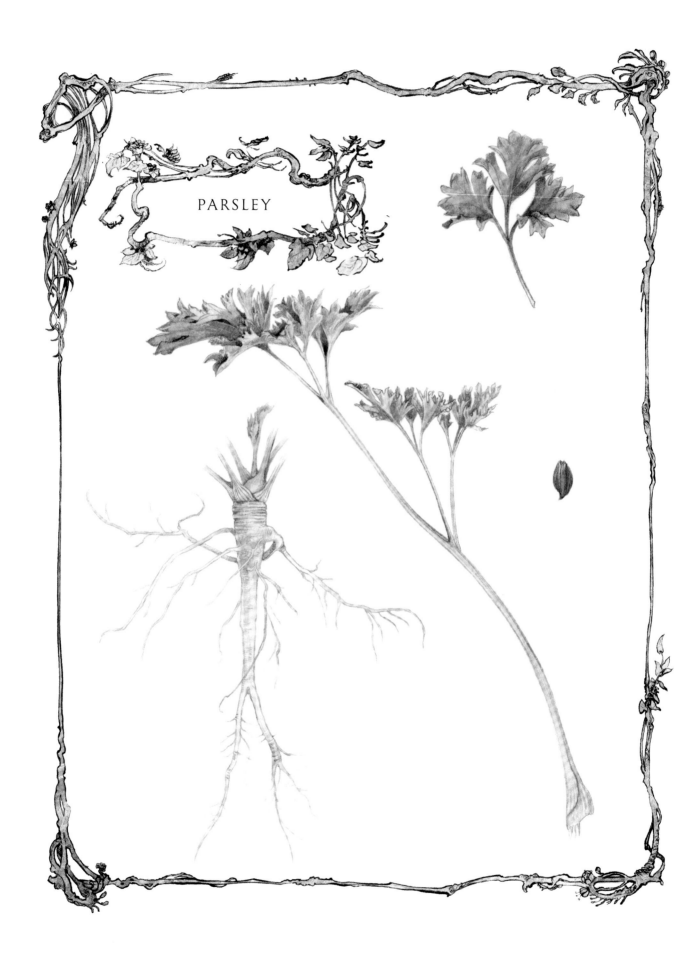

PARSLEY

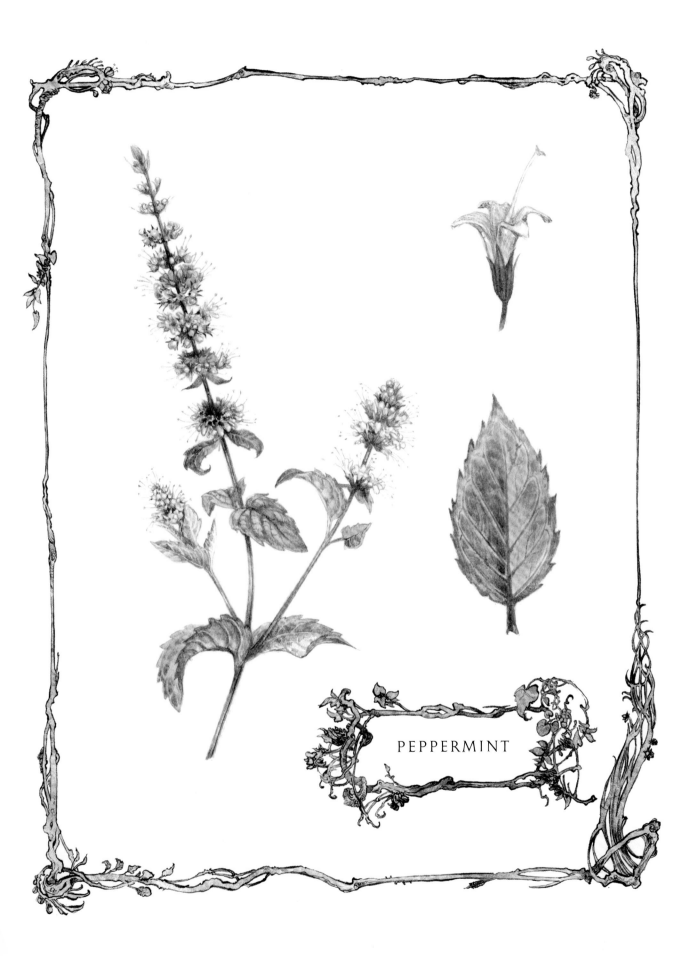

PEPPERMINT

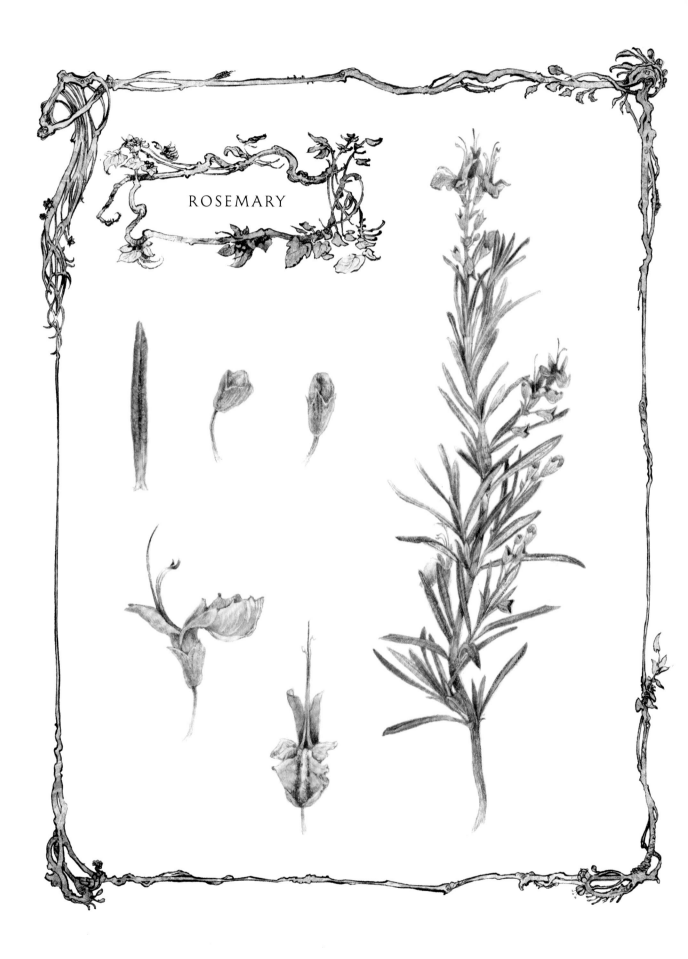

ROSEMARY

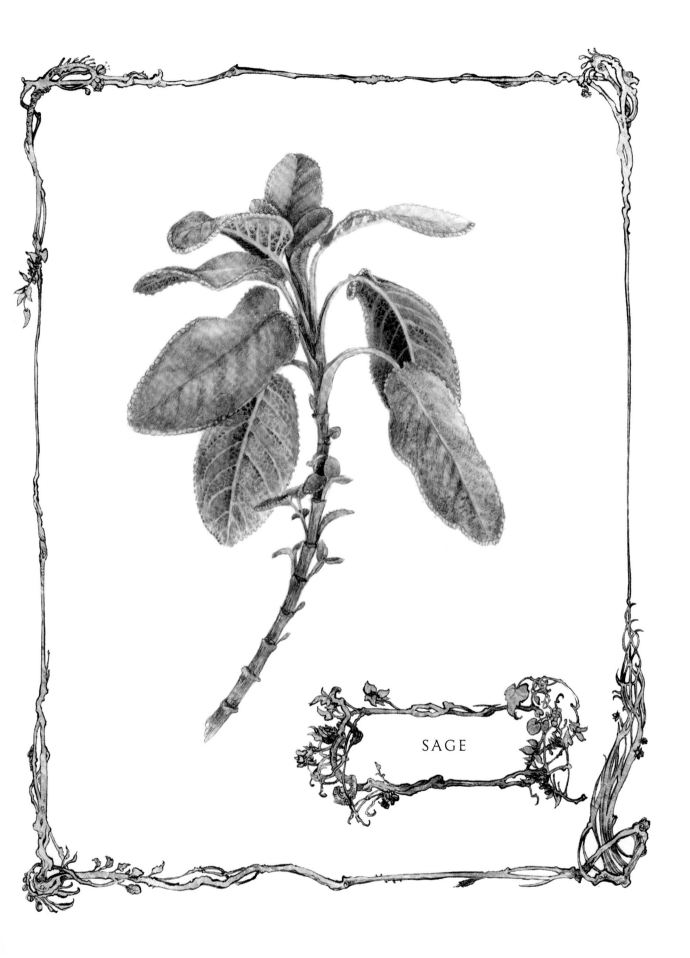

SAGE

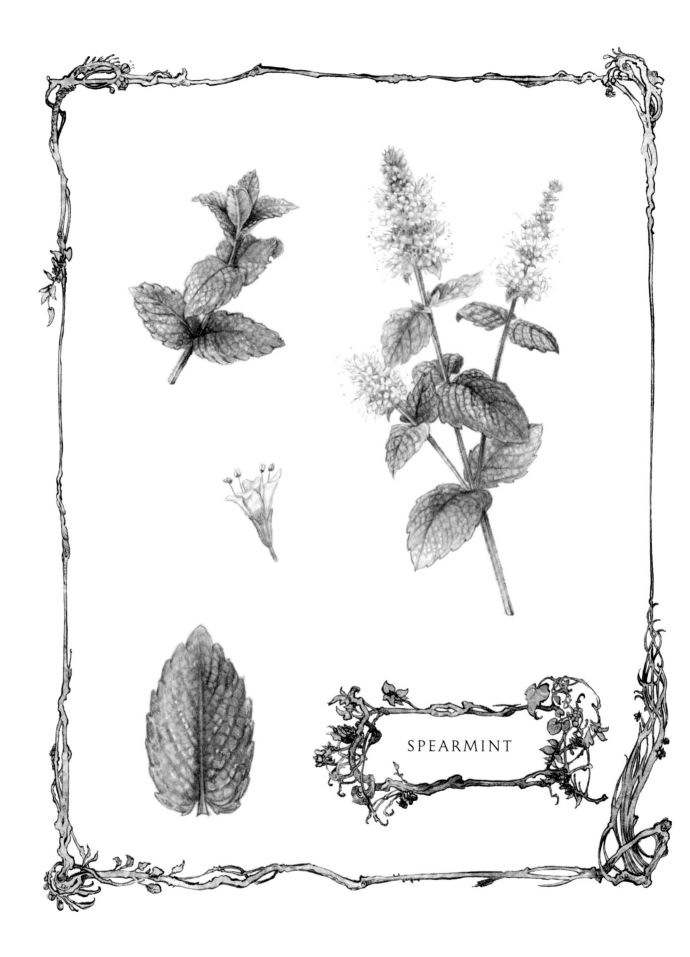

SPEARMINT

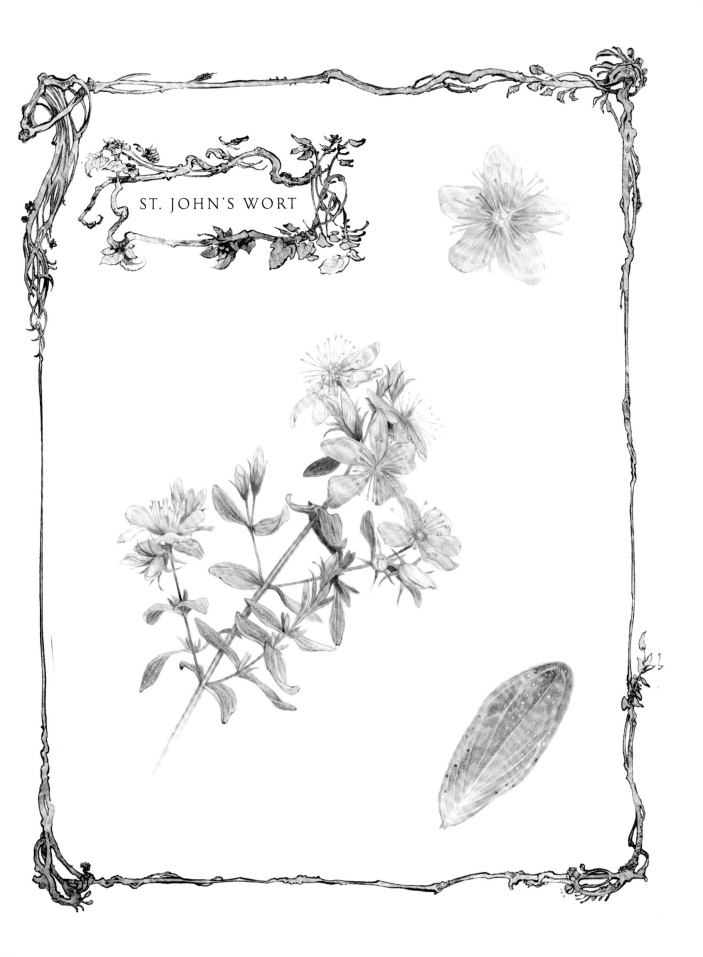

ST. JOHN'S WORT

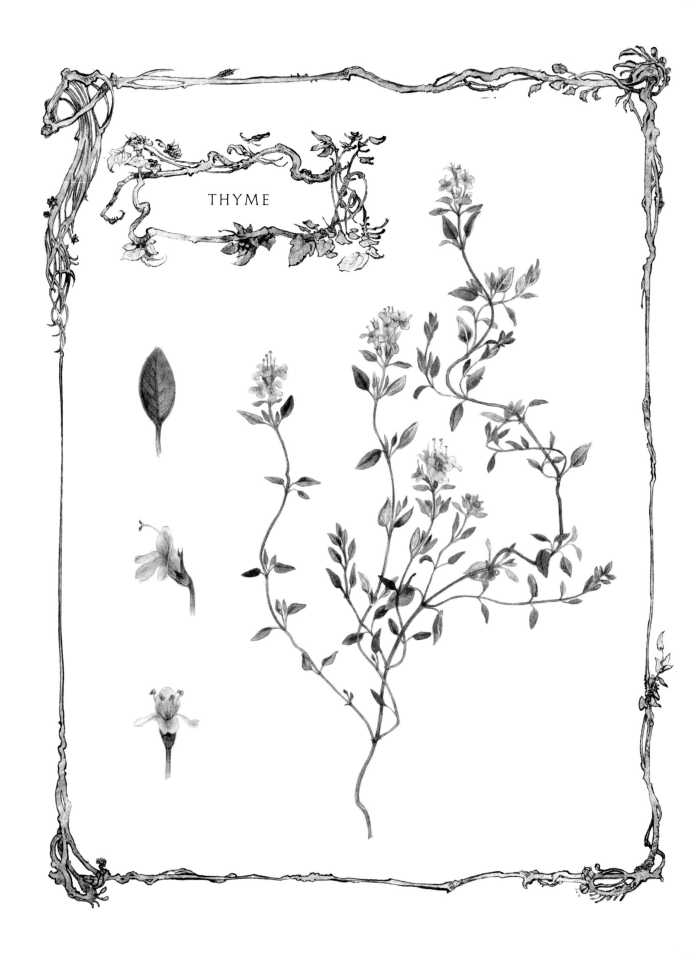

THYME

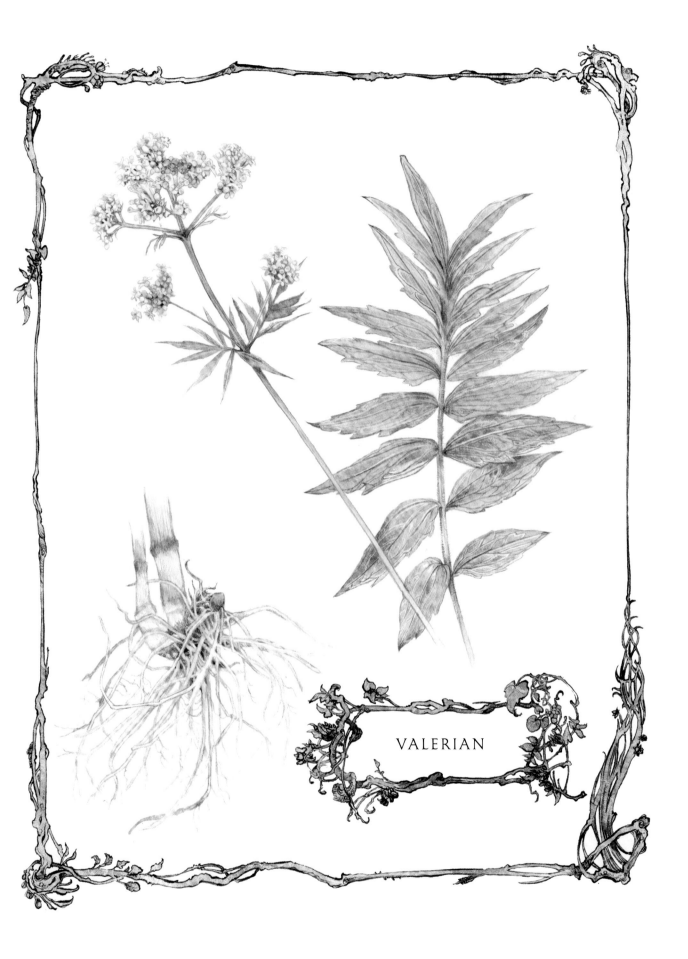

VALERIAN

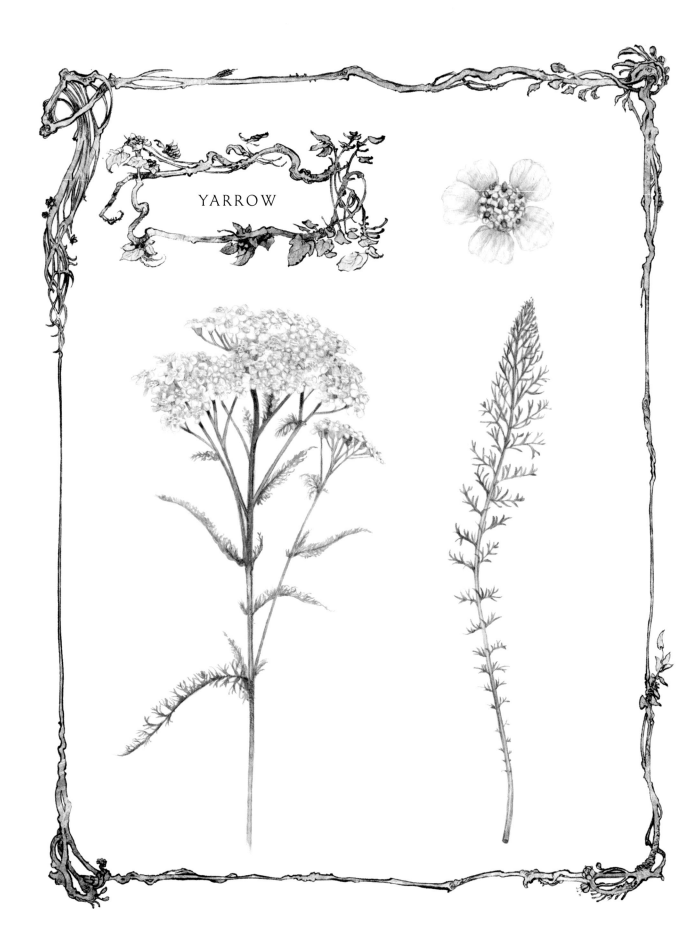

YARROW

GLOSSARY

Acute: A condition or disease with a rapid onset that lasts a short period of time.

Amenorrhea: The absence of menstruation, or one or more missed menstrual periods.

Annual: A plant that completes its life cycle in one year or growing season.

Anorexia *(anorexia nervosa):* An eating disorder in which a person is without an appetite for food and loses more weight than is considered healthy.

Antiseptic: A substance that destroys infection-causing bacteria.

Antiviral: A substance that inhibits the growth of a virus.

Aromatherapy: The therapeutic use of essential oils through scent.

Aromatics: Plants that produce high amounts of essential oil and have strong fragrances.

Arthritis: The inflammation of one or more joints accompanied by pain and stiffness.

Asthma: A chronic lung disease that inflames and narrows the respiratory airways.

Astringent: A substance that dries and contracts organic tissue.

Ayurvedic medicine: A system of healing and health maintenance that originated in India more than three thousand years ago.

Balm: A preparation with a very firm consistency that forms a protective layer on the skin.

Biennial: A plant that completes its life cycle in two or sometimes three years or growing seasons.

Bouquets garnis: A classic culinary combination of bay, parsley, and thyme.

Bulb: The fleshy, underground part of a plant that stores nutrients.

Carrier oil: A fatty plant extraction used for cooking and to dilute essential oils. It is also called a base or a fixed oil.

Catarrh: The inflammation of mucous membranes along with an excessive buildup of mucus in the nose or throat

Chilblains: The painful inflammation of small blood vessels in the skin when exposed to cold and high humidity.

Chinese medicine: Also called Traditional Chinese medicine (TCM), it is a system of healing and health that originated in China several thousand years ago. Many of the remedies are based on herbs.

Chronic: A persistent condition or disease that is long-term.

Cold pressed: A mechanical method for obtaining oil from plant material by pressing it. This is also called expression and expeller pressed.

Colitis: The inflammation of the colon.

Companion planting: The practice of combining mutually beneficial plants within a garden.

Cream: A healing and soothing preparation that is mostly absorbed into the skin.

Crohn's disease: A chronic inflammatory disease of the intestines.

Crown: The upper, above ground part of a root system of a perennial plant.

Cultivar: A variety of plant that is developed and cultivated by humans instead of by natural selection in the wild.

Cutting: A piece of stem, root, or leaf used to propagate a plant.

Decoction: An extraction of medicinal substances made by boiling down the tougher or more fibrous parts of plants such as roots, bark, and seeds.

Dermatitis: A general term that describes the inflammation of the skin when it becomes red, swollen, and sore.

Diuretic: A substance that increases the quantity and flow of urine.

Distillation: A method for extracting essential oil from plant material that uses steam or hot water to separate the water-soluble and non-water-soluble parts of plants.

Eczema: An inflammatory condition that causes areas of the skin to become red, rough, and itchy.

Edema: A painless swelling caused by fluid retention under the skin.

Essential oil: The concentrated, non-water-soluble extraction from plants obtained by distillation or cold pressing. It is also called a volatile oil because it evaporates quickly.

Expectorant: A substance that loosens phlegm and helps to clear the respiratory airways.

Fibromyalgia: A disorder with widespread musculoskeletal pain, fatigue, sleep, memory, and mood issues.

Fines herbes: A classic culinary combination of chervil, chives, parsley, and tarragon.

Flower essence: An infusion of flowers in water, which is then mixed with brandy. It should not be confused with a tincture or essential oil.

Fungal infection: A common infection of the skin caused by a fungus that includes athlete's foot, jock itch, ringworm, and yeast infections.

Gastritis: A condition in which the lining of the stomach is inflamed and irritated.

Gastroenteritis: A condition in which the lining of the stomach and intestines are inflamed and irritated.

Gingivitis: The inflammation of gum tissue.

Gout: A type of arthritis that occurs when uric acid builds up and causes joint inflammation.

Hardening off: The process of conditioning a plant from a protected environment to an outside location.

Hardiness zone: A geographical area defined by its average minimum temperature that is used to determine which plants can be grown there. It is sometimes simply called a zone.

Hemorrhoids: A condition caused by dilated rectal veins. They are also known as piles.

Herbes de Provence: A classic culinary combination of bay, fennel, rosemary, and thyme.

Humus: A form of organic matter that has been broken down to its most basic level.

Hydrosol: Traditionally called floral waters (i.e., rosewater), a hydrosol contains the water-soluble molecules of aromatic plants. It is also called a hydroflorate and hydrolat.

Infusion: An extraction of medicinal substances made by steeping the aerial parts of plants in hot water, or hot or cold oil.

Irritable bowel syndrome (IBS): A disorder that affects the large intestine.

Knot garden: A type of formal garden that is laid out in an intricate, interlacing design.

Liniment: An extraction of medicinal substances from plants made by steeping them in alcohol or witch hazel. It is for external use and should not be confused with a tincture.

Lipophilic: A substance that is not water soluble. It readily combines with or dissolves in lipids or fats. Essential oils are lipophilic.

Loam: Soil that has a balance of sand, silt, and clay.

Lobed: The description of a leaf with deeply indented edges, such as oak or maple tree leaves.

Maceration: An extraction of medicinal substances from plants made by steeping them in cold water.

Mastitis: An infection of breast tissue accompanied by pain, swelling, and redness.

Menorrhagia: A menstrual period with abnormally heavy or prolonged bleeding.

Ointment: A preparation with a slightly firm consistency that forms a protective layer on the skin.

Perennial: A plant that lives for a number of years. The parts above ground often die back in the autumn and come up again in the spring.

Photosensitivity: Heightened sensitivity to sunlight

Pinnate: The description of a leaf that has three or more leaflets on a common stem.

Poultice: A thick, moist paste of plant material that is applied to an affected area of the body.

Premenstrual syndrome (PMS): A term that refers to a wide variety of symptoms that may include mood swings, tender breasts, food cravings, fatigue, irritability, and depression.

Psoriasis: A skin condition that causes itchy or sore patches of thick, red skin accompanied by silvery scales.

Pyorrhea: The inflammation of the sockets of the teeth. It is also known as periodontitis.

Raised bed: A type of garden above the surface of the ground that is contained within a frame.

Raynaud's disease: A disorder of the small blood vessels, usually in the fingers and toes, that causes these areas to feel numb and cool in response to cold temperatures or stress.

Rheumatism: A condition characterized by stiffness and pain in muscles or fibrous tissue, and swelling and pain in the joints.

Rheumatoid arthritis: A type of autoimmune arthritis that causes pain, stiffness, swelling, and limited motion in many joints.

Rhizome: An underground stem that stores nutrients for a plant. It is usually considered as a type of root.

Ringworm: A type of skin infection caused by a fungus.

Salve: A preparation with a semi-firm consistency that forms a protective layer on the skin.

Scabies: A contagious and very itchy skin infection caused by the *Sarcoptes scabiei* mite.

Sciatica: Pain or numbness that runs from the lower back down the leg(s) along the sciatic nerve pathway.

Seasonal affective disorder (SAD): A type of depression that occurs during the same season each year. It most often occurs in winter.

Simples: Preparations that require only one herb rather than a combination of plants.

Sinusitis: The inflammation of the sinuses.

Sitz bath: A method of bathing in which a person sits in shallow water up to the hips. It is also known as a hip bath.

Spike: A long, flower-bearing stem without branches.

Sprain: A stretch and/or tear of a ligament.

Staph infection: An infection caused by the *Staphylococcus* bacteria.

Strain: A stretch and/or tear of a muscle.

Strep throat: A sore throat accompanied by fever that is caused by the *Streptococcus* bacteria.

Sty: An inflamed oil gland on the edge of the eyelid.

Sun tea: A method of making tea by placing herbs in cold water and then setting the container in the sun to brew. It is also known as a solar infusion.

Taproot: The large, main part of a root.

Temporomandibular joint pain (TMJ): A pain that occurs in or near the jaw joint, which is caused by a range of problems.

Tincture: An extraction of medicinal substances from plants made by steeping them in alcohol, vinegar, or cider.

Tisane: A mild infusion often called a tea. Technically, tea is made only from the *Camellia sinensis* plant.

Tonic: An herbal mixture that strengthens and supports a specific system or the entire body.

Toothed: The description of a leaf with jagged edges.

Umbel: The description of a common flower cluster structure with multiple stems radiating from a central stem. Although it can be round like a globe, it most often has the basic shape of an umbrella.

Vaginitis: A medical term used to describe various conditions that cause infection or inflammation of the vagina. It is frequently caused by a fungal infection and called a vaginal yeast infection.

Varicose veins: The name given to enlarged, twisted blood vessels that appear blue and bulging through the skin.

Volatile oil: Another name for essential oil.

Water soluble: A substance that can be dissolved in water.

Yeast infection: A type of fungal infection caused by the overgrowth of yeast.

BIBLIOGRAPHY

Adamson, Melitta Weiss. *Food in Medieval Times*. Westport, CT: Greenwood Press, 2004.

Arrowsmith, Nancy. *Essential Herbal Wisdom: A Complete Exploration of 50 Remarkable Herbs*. Woodbury, MN: Llewellyn Publications, 2009.

Balaban, Naomi E., and James E. Bobick, eds. *The Handy Science Answer Book, Fourth Edition*. Canton, MI: Visible Ink Press, 2011.

Bedson, Paul. *The Complete Family Guide to Natural Healing*. Dingley, Australia: Hinkler Books, 2005.

Binney, Ruth. *The Gardener's Wise Words and Country Ways*. Newton Abbot, England: David and Charles, 2007.

Bird, Stephanie Rose. *Four Seasons of Mojo: An Herbal Guide to Natural Living*. Woodbury, MN: Llewellyn Publications, 2006.

Black, Cynthia. *Natural and Herbal Family Remedies: Storey's Country Wisdom Bulletin A-168*. North Adams, MA: Storey Publishing, 1997.

Bonar, Ann. *Herbs: A Complete Guide to the Cultivation and Use of Wild and Domesticated Herbs*. New York: MacMillan Publishing, 1985.

Bonar, Ann, and Daphne MacCarthy. *How to Grow and Use Herbs*. London: Ward Lock, 1987.

Boxer, Arabella, and Charlotte Parry-Crooke. *The Book of Herbs and Spices*. London: The Hamlyn Publishing Group, 1989.

Brookes, Ian. *Chambers Concise Dictionary*. Edinburgh, Scotland: Chambers Harrap Publishers, 2004.

Campion, Kitty. *The Family Medical Herbal: A Complete Guide to Maintaining Health and Treating Illness with Plants*. New York: Barnes & Noble Books, 1988.

Castleman, Michael. *The Healing Herbs: The Ultimate Guide to the Curative Power of Nature's Medicines*. New York: Bantam Books, 1995.

_____ . *The New Healing Herbs: The Classic Guide to Nature's Best Medicines*. Emmaus, PA: Rodale Press, 2001.

Charles, Denys J. *Antioxidant Properties of Spices, Herbs and Other Sources*. New York: Springer Science and Business Media, 2013.

Chevallier, Andrew. *The Encyclopedia of Medicinal Plants: A Practical Reference Guide to Over 550 Key Herbs and Their Medicinal Uses*. New York: Dorling Kindersley Publishing, 1996.

_____ . *Herbal Remedies*. New York: Dorling Kindersley Publishing, 2007.

Coombes, Allen J. *Dictionary of Plant Names*. Portland, OR: Timber Press, 1985.

Crawford, Amanda McQuade. *Discover Nature's Wonderful Secrets Just for Women*. Roseville, CA: Three Rivers Press, 1997.

Creasy, Rosalind. *The Edible Herb Garden*. North Clarendon, VT: Charles E. Tuttle, 1999.

Crellin, John K., and Jane Philpott. *A Reference Guide to Medicinal Plants: Herbal Medicine Past and Present*. Durham, NC: Duke University Press, 1997.

Culpeper, Nicholas. *Culpeper's Complete Herbal: A Book of Natural Remedies for Ancient Ills*. Ware, England: Wordsworth Editions, 1995.

Cumo, Christopher. *Encyclopedia of Cultivated Plants: From Acacia to Zinnia, Volume 1*. Santa Barbara, CA: ABC-CLIO, 2013.

Curtis, Susan, and Louise Green. *Home Herbal: The Ultimate Guide to Cooking, Brewing, and Blending Your Own Herbs*. New York: Dorling Kindersley Publishing, 2011.

D'Andrea, Jeanne. *Ancient Herbs in the J. Paul Getty Museum Gardens*. Malibu, CA: J. Paul Getty Museum, 1989.

Damrosch, Barbara, and Regina Ryan. *The Garden Primer: The Completely Revised Gardener's Bible*. New York: Workman Publishing, 2008.

Dobelis, Inge N., ed. *Magic and Medicine of Plants*. Pleasantville, NY: The Reader's Digest Association, 1986.

Duke, James A. *The Green Pharmacy*. Emmaus, PA: Rodale Press, 1997.

Durkin, Philip. *The Oxford Guide to Etymology*. New York: Oxford University Press, 2009.

Eastman, John Andrew. *The Book of Field and Roadside: Open-country Weeds, Trees, and Wildflowers of Eastern North America*. Mechanicsburg, PA: Stackpole Books, 2003.

Foster, Steven, and Rebecca L. Johnson. *National Geographic Desk Reference to Nature's Medicine*. Washington, DC: National Geographic Society, 2008.

Garland, Sarah. *The Complete Book of Herbs and Spices*. London: Frances Lincoln, 2004.

_____ . *The Herb Garden*. London: Frances Lincoln, 2006.

Gilbertie, Sal, and Larry Sheehan. *Herb Gardening from the Ground Up: Everything You Need to Know About Growing Your Favorite Herbs*. New York: Ten Speed Press, 2012.

Gladstar, Rosemary. *Herbal Healing for Women*. New York: Fireside, 1993.

_____ . *Medicinal Herbs: A Beginner's Guide*. North Adams, MA: Storey Publishing, 2012.

Grieve, Margaret. *A Modern Herbal, Volumes I and II*. Mineola, NY: Dover Publications, 1971.

Griggs, Barbara. *The Home Herbal: A Handbook of Simple Remedies*. London: Robert Hale, 1986.

Griggs, Barbara, and Barbara Van der Zee. *Green Pharmacy: The History and Evolution of Western Herbal Medicine*. Rochester, VT: Healing Arts Press, 1997.

Heilmeyer, Marina. *Ancient Herbs*. Los Angeles, CA: Getty Publications, 2007.

Jain, Narendra. *Ayurvedic and Herbal Remedies for Arthritis*. New Delhi, India: Pustak Mahal, 2006.

Kamhi, Ellen. *Alternative Medicine Magazine's Definitive Guide to Weight Loss: 10 Healthy Way to Permanently Shed Unwanted Pounds, Second Edition*. Berkeley, CA: Celestial Arts, 2007.

Kelly, Kate. *Early Civilizations: Prehistoric Times to 500 C.E.* New York: Facts on File, 2009.

Kennedy, David O. *Plants and the Human Brain*. New York: Oxford University Press, 2014.

Kloss, Jethro. *Back to Eden: A Human Interest Story of Health and Restoration to be Found in Herb, Root, and Bark, Second Edition*. Twin Lakes, WI: Lotus Press, 1999.

Kowalchik, Claire, and William H. Hylton, eds. *Rodale's Illustrated Encyclopedia of Herbs*. Emmaus, PA: Rodale Press, 1998.

Kress, Stephen W. *The Bird Garden*. New York: Dorling Kindersley Publishing, 1995.

Lawless, Julia. *The Complete Illustrated Guide to Aromatherapy: A Practical Approach to the Use of Essential Oils for Health and Well-Being*. London: Element Books, 1999.

_____ . *The Illustrated Encyclopedia of Essential Oils: The Complete Guide to the Use of Oils in Aromatherapy and Herbalism*. London: Element Books, 1995.

Leyel, C. F. *Herbal Delights*. Pomeroy, WA: Health Research, 2007.

Libster, Martha. *Delmar's Integrative Herb Guide for Nurses*. Independence, KY: Cengage Learning, 2001.

Mabey, Richard, and Michael McIntyre. *The New Age Herbalist: How to Use Herbs for Healing, Nutrition, Body Care and Relaxation*. New York: Fireside Books, 1988.

Marchese, C. Marina, and Kim Flottum. *The Honey Connoisseur*. New York: Black Dog & Leventhal Publishers, 2013.

Martin, Ingrid. *Aromatherapy for Massage Practitioners*. Baltimore: Lippincott Williams & Wilkins, 2007.

Mayer, Dale. *The Complete Guide to Companion Planting: Everything You Need to Know to Make Your Garden Successful*. Ocala, FL: Atlantic Publishing Group, 2010.

McBride, Kami. *The Herbal Kitchen: 50 Easy-to-Find Herbs and Over 250 Recipes to Bring Lasting Health to Your Family*. San Francisco: Conari Press, 2010.

McIntyre, Anne. *Drink to Your Health: Delicious Juices, Teas, Soups, and Smoothies that Help You Look and Feel Great*. New York: Fireside, 2000.

McLeod, Judyth A. *In a Unicorn's Garden: Recreating the Mystery and Magic of Medieval Gardens*. London: Murdoch Books UK, 2008.

McVicar, Jekka. *Grow Herbs: An Inspiring Guide to Growing and Using Herbs*. New York: Dorling Kindersley Publishing, 2010.

Mitchell, Deborah. *The Family Guide to Vitamins, Herbs, and Supplements*. New York: St. Martin's Press, 2011.

Neal, Bill. *Gardener's Latin: A Lexicon*. Chapel Hill, NC: Algonquin Books of Chapel Hill, 1992.

Newman, Paul B. *Daily Life in the Middle Ages*. Jefferson, NC: McFarland & Company, 2001.

Norman, Jill. *Salad Herbs: How to Grow and Use Them in the Kitchen*. London: Dorling Kindersley Publishing, 1989.

Nunn, John F. *Ancient Egyptian Medicine*. Norman, OK: University of Oklahoma Press, 1996.

Ogden, Ellen Ecker. *The Complete Kitchen Garden: An Inspired Collection of Garden Designs and 100 Seasonal Recipes*. New York: Stewart, Tabori & Chang, 2011.

Philbrick, John, and Helen Philbrick. *Gardening for Health and Nutrition: An Introduction to the Method of Biodynamic Gardening*. Hudson, NY: Anthroposophic Press, 1988.

Pizzorno, Joseph E., and Michael T. Murray, eds. *Textbook of Natural Medicine, Fourth Edition*. St. Louis, MO: Elsevier, 2013.

Price, Shirley. *Aromatherapy for Common Ailments*. New York: Fireside, 1991.

Raghavan, Susheela. *Handbook of Spices, Seasonings, and Flavorings, Second Edition*. Boca Raton, FL: CRC Press, 2007.

Riotte, Louise. *Roses Love Garlic: Companion Planting and Other Secrets of Flowers, Second Edition*. North Adams, MA: Storey Publishing, 1998.

Robertson, Ian. *Six Thousand Years Up the Garden Path: An Exceptional Journey*. Bloomington, IN: iUniverse, 2010.

Rose, Jeanne. *375 Essential Oils and Hydrosols*. Berkeley, CA: Frog Books, 1999.

Russell, Tracy, and Catherine Abbott, eds. *The Green Smoothie Garden: Grow Your Own Produce for the Most Nutritious Green Smoothie Recipes Possible!* Avon, MA: Adams Media, 2014.

Schiller, Carol, and David Schiller. *The Aromatherapy Encyclopedia: A Concise Guide to Over 385 Plant Oils.* Laguna Beach, CA: Basic Health Publications, 2008.

Shababy, Doreen. *The Wild and Weedy Apothecary: An A to Z Book of Herbal Concoctions, Recipes & Remedies, Practical Know How & Food for the Soul.* Woodbury, MN: Llewellyn Publications, 2010.

Shaudys, Phyllis. *The Pleasure of Herbs: A Month-by-Month Guide to Growing, Using, and Enjoying Herbs.* Pownal, VT: Storey Communications, 1986.

Shealy, C. Norman. *The Healing Remedies Sourcebook: Over 1,000 Natural Remedies to Prevent and Cure Common Ailments.* Boston: Da Capo Press, 2012.

Small, Ernest. *Culinary Herbs, Second Edition.* Ottawa, Canada: National Research Council of Canada, 2006.

Smith, Miranda. *Your Backyard Herb Garden: A Gardener's Guide to Growing Over 50 Herbs.* Emmaus, PA: Rodale Press, 1997.

Solomon, Steve. *Gardening When It Counts: Growing Food in Hard Times.* Gabriola Island, Canada: New Society Publishers, 2013.

Sonnedecker, Glenn. *The History of Pharmacy.* Philadelphia, PA: J. B. Lippincott, 1976.

Starcher, Allison Mia. *Good Bugs for Your Garden.* Chapel Hill, NC: Algonquin Books of Chapel Hill, 1998.

Staub, Jack. *75 Exceptional Herbs for Your Garden.* Layton, UT: Gibbs Smith, 2008.

Stearns, Raymond Phineas. *Science in the British Colonies of America.* Champaign, IL: University of Illinois Press, 1970.

Steel, Susannah, ed. *Home Herbal: Cook, Brew, and Blend Your Own Herbs.* New York: Dorling Kindersley Publishing, 2011.

Swindells, Philip. *The Harlow Car Book of Herb Gardening.* Newton Abbot, England: David and Charles, 1988.

Tierra, Lesley. *Healing with the Herbs of Life.* New York: Crossing Press, 2003.

Tucker, Arthur O., and Thomas Debaggio. *The Encyclopedia of Herbs: A Comprehensive Reference to Herbs of Flavor and Fragrance.* Portland, OR: Timber Press, 2009.

Varney, Bill, and Sylvia Varney. *Herbs: Growing and Using the Plants of Romance.* Littleton, CO: Ironwood Press, 1998.

Vaughan, J. G., and P. A. Judd. *The Oxford Book of Health Foods: A Comprehensive Guide to Natural Remedies.* New York: Oxford University Press, 2003.

Vincent, Wendy. *The Complete Guide to Growing Healing and Medicinal Herbs: A Complete Step-by-Step Guide*. Ocala, FL: Atlantic Publishing Group, 2011.

Watson, Franzesca. *Aromatherapy Blends and Remedies*. London: Thorsons, 1995.

Wheelwright, Edith Grey. *Medicinal Plants and Their History*. New York: Dover Publications, 1974.

Wilson, Roberta. *Aromatherapy*. New York: Penguin Putnam, 2002.

Worwood, Valerie Ann. *The Complete Book of Essential Oils and Aromatherapy*. San Rafael, CA: New World Library, 1991.

Yeager, Selene. *The Doctors Book of Food Remedies*. Emmaus, PA: Rodale Press, 2008.

Online Resources

Hive and Honey Apiary. "The Honey Bee." Paisley, Ontario, Canada. Accessed July 15, 2014. http://www.hiveandhoneyapiary.com.

USDA Plant Hardiness Zone Map, 2012. Agricultural Research Service, US Department of Agriculture. Accessed August 1, 2014. http://planthardiness.ars.usda.gov.

WebMD. New York. Accessed throughout 2014. http://www.webmd.com.

INDEX

To Write to the Author

If you wish to contact the author or would like more information about this book, please write to the author in care of Llewellyn Worldwide Ltd. and we will forward your request. Both the author and publisher appreciate hearing from you and learning of your enjoyment of this book and how it has helped you. Llewellyn Worldwide Ltd. cannot guarantee that every letter written to the author can be answered, but all will be forwarded. Please write to:

Sandra Kynes
℅ Llewellyn Worldwide
2143 Wooddale Drive
Woodbury, MN 55125-2989

Please enclose a self-addressed stamped envelope for reply,
or $1.00 to cover costs. If outside the U.S.A., enclose
an international postal reply coupon.

Many of Llewellyn's authors have websites with additional information and resources.
For more information, please visit our website at http://www.llewellyn.com.